V VETERINARY

M MEDICAL

S SCHOOL

A ADMISSION

R REQUIREMENTS

VETERINARY MEDICAL SCHOOL ADMISSION REQUIREMENTS

2013 Edition for 2014 Matriculation

Association of American
Veterinary Medical Colleges

PURDUE UNIVERSITY PRESS   WEST LAFAYETTE, INDIANA

Compiled by the Association of American Veterinary Medical Colleges;
Shaba Lightfoot, editor

Cover photograph courtesy of the University of Pennsylvania
Back cover photographs courtesy of:
1. Courtesy of the University of Wisconsin
2. Courtesy of Washington State University

Printed in the United States of America

Paperback ISBN: 978-155753-645-7
ePub ISBN: 978-1-61249-264-3
ePDF ISBN: 978-1-61249-263-6
ISSN: 1089-6465

CONTENTS

FOREWORD

These are exciting times for veterinary medicine. As you read these words, you are taking your first steps toward entering a profession that bridges animal, human and ecosystem health. The veterinary medical profession offers a variety of exciting, enriching, and fulfilling career choices, including companion animal medicine, food animal medicine, public health, laboratory animal medicine, basic biomedical research, and more. We understand that getting started and making sense of all the choices and requirements can be challenging, but you've come to the right place by accessing this *Veterinary Medical School Admission Requirements (VMSAR)* publication, which provides the essential information you need to begin your journey.

The Association of American Veterinary Medical Colleges (AAVMC) is pleased to provide this publication, which outlines the application procedures and processes of our member colleges. All of the veterinary colleges and schools highlighted in this publication are accredited by the American Veterinary Medical Association or engaged in the accreditation process.

Published annually, VMSAR helps prospective students understand and consider the many important factors that come into play when preparing for an education in veterinary medicine, including cost, financial aid, potential debt, special programs, standardized tests, the AAVMC Veterinary Medical College Application Service (VMCAS), and the various colleges' and schools' residency admissions requirements.

VMSAR also provides current-year information on application requirements for all AAVMC member institutions. This information, presented in an easy-to-understand format, helps applicants determine their best choices for submitting successful applications. Often, an applicant's state of residence will play a major role in admissions, so that's a good place to begin. Adhering to the pre-veterinary medical course requirements in your state of residence makes fulfilling the requirements more time-effective and easier to manage.

As is the case with other health professions, the pursuit and achievement of a veterinary medical education represents a considerable investment of your time, effort and financial resources. If cost is an overriding concern, cost-saving strategies include focusing on in-state veterinary medical schools or states that offer in-state tuition as part of special agreements with neighboring states. Other strategies include focusing on areas of greatest need, such as rural veterinary practice where loan repayment options might be available, or considering additional training that often provides greater compensation. Additional training might also include post-graduate work that could lead to a faculty position in higher education or a career as a research scientist with biological, food, and pharmaceutical companies, or governmental agencies. There are 43 specialties in veterinary medicine or discipline-based graduate training programs to consider, including surgery, neurology, pathology, and more.

There are many details and choices to contemplate and process, but rest assured that you've chosen to pursue a career in a noble and well-respected profession, one that will prepare you to make important contributions to society at the intersection of animal, human and ecosystem health.

More information can be found on individual college and school websites or on the AAVMC website at www.aavmc.org. Prospective students can also contact the appropriate admissions office at each school or the VMCAS Student and Advisor Hotline, either by email (vmcasinfo@vmcas.org) or by calling VMCAS at (617) 612-2884.

The AAVMC extends best wishes to all who desire to pursue a career in veterinary medicine. Society holds veterinarians in high esteem because of the significant contributions they make in improving the health and wellbeing of the people and animals they serve and because of the unique role that veterinarians play in fostering the human/animal bond.

Perhaps no other medical career provides such a broad base of biomedical training and leads to so many different areas of practice. In my own case, a veterinary medical education has enabled me to fulfill a variety of roles, including service as an officer in the United States Air Force, work in a mixed animal practice, in public health as an official with the U.S. Centers for Disease Control and Prevention, and now, as executive director of the AAVMC.

All of us at the AAVMC wish you well in your pursuit of a veterinary medical education and commend your decision to acquire the training and the understanding you need to practice in this extraordinary and rewarding profession.

Dr. Andrew Maccabe
AAVMC Executive Director

About the AAVMC

The Association of American Veterinary Medical Colleges (AAVMC) is a non-profit membership organization working to protect and improve the health and welfare of animals, people, and the environment by advancing academic veterinary medicine. The association was founded in 1966 by the deans of the then-existing 18 colleges of veterinary medicine in the United States and three in Canada. During the 1970s and 1980s, AAVMC's membership expanded to include departments of veterinary science in colleges of agriculture, and in the 1990s to include divisions or departments of comparative medicine. In 2008, AAVMC began accepting non-accredited colleges and schools of veterinary medicine as affiliate members.

Today, AAVMC provides leadership for an academic veterinary medical community which includes all 28 colleges of veterinary medicine in the United States; nine departments of veterinary science; nine departments of comparative medicine; all five veterinary medical colleges in Canada; 12 accredited colleges of veterinary medicine in Australia, Grenada, Ireland, Mexico, the Netherlands, New Zealand, St. Kitts, and the United Kingdom, and four affiliate members.

Mission

AAVMC provides leadership for and promotes excellence in academic veterinary medicine to prepare the veterinary workforce with the scientific knowledge and skills required to meet societal needs through the protection of animal health, the relief of animal suffering, the conservation of animal resources, the promotion of public health, and the advancement of medical knowledge. AAVMC pursues its mission by providing leadership in:

- Advocating on behalf of academic veterinary medicine;
- Serving as a catalyst and convener on issues of importance to academic veterinary medicine;
- Providing information, knowledge and solutions to support members' work;
- Facilitating enrollment in veterinary medical schools and colleges; and
- Building global partnerships and coalitions to advance our collective goals.

Strategic Goals

1. Lead efforts to review, evaluate, and improve veterinary medical education in order to prepare graduates with the competencies needed to address societal needs.

2. Lead efforts to increase the amount of veterinary research conducted and the number of graduates entering research careers.
3. Lead efforts to recruit a student body aligned with the demands for veterinary expertise.
4. Lead efforts to increase the number of racially and/or ethnically underrepresented in veterinary medicine (*URVM) individuals throughout academic veterinary medicine.
5. Lead efforts to develop the next generation of leaders for academic veterinary medicine.
6. Strengthen AAVMC's capacity to better serve its members, partners, and other stakeholders in advancing the AAVMC mission.

*"URVMs are populations of individuals whose advancement in the veterinary medical profession have historically been disproportionately impacted by six specific aspects of diversity (gender, race, ethnicity, and geographic, socio-economic, and educational disadvantage) due to legal, cultural or social climate impediments." *Definition of Underrepresented in Veterinary Medicine (URVM)*, approved by the AAVMC Board of Directors, July 20, 2008.

VETERINARY MEDICINE: OPPORTUNITIES AND CHOICES

Veterinarians help animals and people live longer, healthier lives. They serve society through the protection of animal health and welfare, the prevention and relief of animal suffering, the conservation of animal resources, the promotion of public health, and the advancement of medical knowledge. The Doctor of Veterinary Medicine degree can lead to diverse career opportunities and different lifestyles from a solo mixed-animal practice in a rural area to a teaching or research position at an urban university, medical center, or industrial laboratory. The majority of veterinarians in the United States are in private clinical practice, although significant numbers are involved in preventive medicine, regulatory veterinary medicine, military veterinary medicine, laboratory animal medicine, research and development in industry, and teaching and research in a variety of basic science and clinical disciplines.

The Spectrum of Opportunities in Veterinary Medicine

Veterinarians may choose to become specialists in a clinical area or to work with particular species. The first step on the path toward specialization is usually an internship.

1) Further Training

Internship

Internships are 1-year programs in either small- or large-animal medicine and surgery. The most prestigious internship programs are at veterinary medical colleges or at very large private veterinary hospitals with board-certified veterinarians on staff. Since internships are usually at large referral centers, interns are exposed to a larger number of challenging cases than they would be likely to see in a smaller private practice.

Veterinary students in their senior year and veterinary graduates apply for internships through a matching program. Internship applicants and training hospitals rank each other in order of preference, and a computerized system matches each applicant with the highest-ranking teaching hospital that ranked the applicant. Academic performance in the veterinary professional curriculum, as well as recommendations from veterinary school faculty, is considered in the ranking of internship applicants.

Most veterinary interns in the United States receive a nominal salary, and their educational debts, if any, may be postponed in some governmentally subsidized loan programs. Veterinarians can sometimes command a higher starting salary in private practice after completion of an internship. Also, an internship is often the next step, after receiving the veterinary degree, toward residency and board certification.

Residency Training

Residency training is more specialized than an internship. Residency training programs are competitive and most require that the prospective residents complete an internship or equivalent private-practice experience prior to beginning the residency programs. Residency training is available in disciplines as varied as internal medicine, surgery, preventive medicine, behavior, toxicology, dentistry, and pathology.

The programs take 2 to 3 years to complete, depending on the nature of the specialty. Successful completion of a residency often is an important step toward attainment of board certification. Some residencies combine research and graduate study leading to master's or PhD degrees.

Board Certification

Currently, there are 22 AVMA-recognized veterinary specialty organizations comprising of 40 distinct specialties: anesthesiology, animal behavior, clinical pharmacology, dentistry, dermatology, emergency and critical care, internal medicine, laboratory animal medicine, microbiology, nutrition, ophthalmology, pathology, poultry medicine, private practice, preventive medicine, radiology, surgery, sports medicine and rehabilitation, theriogenology (reproduction), toxicology, and zoological medicine. Veterinarians may become board certified by completing rigorous postgraduate training, education, and examination requirements.

2) Private and Public Practice

The majority of veterinary graduates are engaged in private practice, either as an owner of a solo practice or, more likely, as a partner or associate in a group practice. Increasingly, veterinarians work together as a team, which allows a wider range of services to be provided.

Small-animal veterinarians focus their efforts primarily on dogs and cats but are seeing a growing number of other pets, including other small mammals, birds, reptiles, and fish.

Large animal veterinarians often place their emphasis on horses, cattle, or pigs, and work both on a farm-call and an in-clinic basis. A mixed-animal veterinarian works with all types of domestic animals.

Public practice provides a variety of opportunities at the international, national, state, county, or city levels. There are exciting career opportunities for veterinarians in food safety, public health, the military, animal disease control and research. Some veterinarians are employed by zoos and aquariums, wildlife conservation groups, game farms, or fisheries.

3) Industry

Veterinarians have many opportunities available to them in private industry, particularly in the fields of nutrition and pharmaceuticals. Assisting in the development of new products in the animal industry, conducting research for pharmaceutical companies, diagnosing disease and drug effects as pathologists, or safeguarding the health of laboratory animal colonies are all interesting career possibilities.

4) Conclusion

By the very nature of the comparative medical education that veterinarians receive, the many species of animals they care for and work for, and the wide variety of clientele served, the opportunities available to today's veterinarian are abundant.

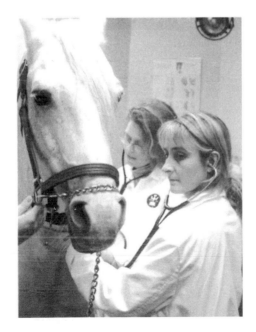

A Tufts University Cummings School of Veterinary Medicine student checks out a horse with advice from her professor. Photo courtesy of Andy Cunningham of the Tufts University Cummings School of Veterinary Medicine.

AAVMC Member Institutions and the Role of Accreditation

Veterinary Schools join the AAVMC as institutional or affiliate members. A key difference between these two membership categories is whether a college/school of veterinary medicine is accredited by the American Veterinary Medical Association's Council on Education (AVMA/COE). Only AVMA/COE accredited colleges of veterinary medicine may join AAVMC as an institutional (voting) member. Colleges of veterinary medicine that are not AVMA-accredited may join AAVMC as an affiliate member (non-voting) only. Several of AAVMC's affiliate members (Non-AVMA/COE accredited institutions) have entered into agreements with AAVMC institutional members for clinical training. It is important for prospective veterinary students to know the different implications of attending and/or graduating from AVMA/COE accredited vs. non-AVMA/COE accredited colleges of veterinary medicine as it pertains to educational options and eventually seeking and obtaining a license to practice veterinary medicine. AAVMC encourages its affiliate members to become AVMA/COE accredited.

Accreditation

The AVMA/COE accredits DVM or equivalent educational programs. Accreditation through the AVMA/COE assures that minimum standards in veterinary medical education are met by accredited colleges of veterinary medicine and that students enrolled in these colleges receive an education that will prepare them for entry-level positions in the profession. In the United States, graduation from an AVMA/COE accredited college of veterinary medicine is an important pre-requisite for application for licensure. Internationally, some veterinary schools have chosen to seek AVMA/COE accreditation in addition to accreditation by the competent authority in their own regions. AVMA/COE accreditation of international veterinary schools provides assurance that those programs of education meet the same standards as other similarly accredited schools.

Additionally, AVMA/COE accreditation assures:
- Prospective students that they will meet a competency threshold for entry into practice, including eligibility for professional credentialing and/or licensure;
- Employers that graduates have achieved specified learning goals and are prepared to begin professional practice;

- Faculty, deans, and administrators that their programs measure satisfactorily against national standards and their own stated missions and goals;
- The public that public health and safety concerns are being addressed; and
- The veterinary profession that the science and art of veterinary medicine are being advanced through contemporary curricula.

*Source: The source for this information and a site recommended for obtaining additional information is the following website: http://www.avma.org/education/cvea/about_accred.asp

Licensure

Licensure in the United States

In the United States, requirements for licensure are set by individual state regulatory boards. The North American Veterinary Licensing Exam (NAVLE) and any additional state exams must be taken by a graduate to become eligible for state licensure. The NAVLE, which is administered by the National Board of Veterinary Medical Examiners (NBVME), fulfills a core requirement for licensure to practice veterinary medicine in all jurisdictions in the United States and Canada. Mexico does not require NAVLE. In addition to the NAVLE, state regulatory boards will have other licensure requirements, which may include state-specific examinations.

To be eligible to take the NAVLE, applicants must have graduated from either an AVMA/COE- accredited college of veterinary medicine or a non-AVMA/COE accredited college (see following details).

Applicants who graduated from a non-AVME/COE accredited college must also have a certification of eligibility, which can come from one of two sources: the Educational Commission for Foreign Veterinary Graduates (ECFVG) Certification Program (http://www.avma.org/education/ecfvg/default.asp) or the Program for the Assessment of Veterinary Education Equivalence (PAVE) (http://www.aavsb.org/PAVE/PAVE Home.aspx).

All state regulatory boards accept the ECFVG certification, administered through the AVMA, as meeting in full or in part the educational prerequisite for licensure eligibility. At this time, 28 state regulatory boards also accept PAVE certification, which is administered through the American Association of Veterinary State Boards (AAVSB).

It is important to note that prerequisites for licensure eligibility and requirements for licensure vary amongst state regulatory boards and are subject to periodic modification.

Licensure Outside the United States

Mutual recognition arrangements apply to jurisdictions where there are AVMA/COE accredited schools. These specify that graduates of AVMA/COE accredited schools in the United States and Canada are permitted to obtain licensure to practice under terms no less favorable than graduates of schools accredited by the competent authority in that jurisdiction.

DECIDING WHERE TO APPLY

There are several factors, as well as the issue of accreditation, that an applicant must consider in identifying school(s) to submit an application for admissions. In addition to licensure issues, there may be economic, educational options, or other differences that students should consider in making decisions on where to apply. This book is intended to provide important information about AAVMC members to assist in informed decision-making for students considering applying to one or more veterinary colleges.

Geographical Listing of AAVMC Institutional (AVMA/ COE Accredited) Veterinary Schools and Directory of Admissions Offices

United States

Alabama
Auburn University
Office for Academic Affairs
College of Veterinary Medicine
217 Goodwin/Overton
Auburn AL 36849-5536

Tuskegee University
Office of Admissions and Recruitment
School of Veterinary Medicine
100 Dr. Frederick Patterson Hall
Tuskegee AL 36088

California
University of California
School of Veterinary Medicine
Office of the Dean-Student Programs
One Shields Avenue
Davis CA 95616

Western University of Health Sciences
Office of Admissions
College of Veterinary Medicine
309 East 2nd Street
Pomona CA 91766-1854

Colorado
Colorado State University
College of Veterinary Medicine and
    Biomedical Sciences
1601 Campus Delivery – Office of the
    Dean
Fort Collins CO 80523-1601

Florida
University of Florida
Admissions Office
College of Veterinary Medicine
P.O. Box 100125
Gainesville FL 32610-0125

Georgia
The University of Georgia
Admissions Department
Office for Academic Affairs
College of Veterinary Medicine
Athens GA 30602-7372

Illinois
University of Illinois
College of Veterinary Medicine
Office of Academic and Student Affairs
2001 South Lincoln Avenue,
    Room 2271g
Urbana IL 61802

Indiana
Purdue University
Student Services Center
College of Veterinary Medicine
625 Harrison Street
West Lafayette IN 47907-2026

Iowa
Iowa State University
Office of Admissions
College of Veterinary Medicine
2270 Veterinary Medicine
P.O. Box 3020
Ames IA 50010-3020

7

Kansas
Kansas State University
Office of Admissions
College of Veterinary Medicine
101 Trotter Hall
Manhattan KS 66506-5601

Louisiana
Louisiana State University
Office of Student and Academic Affairs
School of Veterinary Medicine
Skip Bertman Drive
Baton Rouge LA 70803

Massachusetts
Tufts University
Office of Admissions
Cummings School of Veterinary
   Medicine
200 Westboro Road
North Grafton MA 01536

Michigan
Michigan State University
Office of Admissions
College of Veterinary Medicine
784 Wilson Road
F-110 Veterinary Medical Center
East Lansing MI 48824

Minnesota
University of Minnesota
Office of Academic and Student Affairs
College of Veterinary Medicine
108 Pomeroy Center
1964 Fitch Ave.
St. Paul MN 55108

Mississippi
Mississippi State University
Office of Student Admissions
College of Veterinary Medicine
P.O. Box 6100
Mississippi State MS 39762

Missouri
University of Missouri-Columbia
Office of Academic Affairs
College of Veterinary Medicine
W203 Veterinary Medicine Building
Columbia MO 65211

New York
Cornell University
Office of Student & Academic Services
College of Veterinary Medicine
S2-009 Schurman Hall
Ithaca NY 14853-6401

North Carolina
North Carolina State University
Student Services Office
College of Veterinary Medicine
1060 William Moore Drive, Box 8401
Raleigh NC 27607

Ohio
The Ohio State University
Office of Student Affairs
College of Veterinary Medicine
Suite 127 Veterinary Medicine
   Academic Building
1900 Coffey Road
Columbus OH 43210-1089

Oklahoma
Oklahoma State University
Office of Admissions
112 McElroy Hall
Center for Veterinary Health Sciences
College of Veterinary Medicine
Stillwater OK 74078-2003

Oregon
Oregon State University
Office of the Dean
Attention: Admissions
College of Veterinary Medicine
200 Magruder Hall
Corvallis OR 97331-4801

Pennsylvania
University of Pennsylvania
Admissions Office
School of Veterinary Medicine
3800 Spruce Street
Philadelphia PA 19104-6044

Tennessee
The University of Tennessee
Admissions Office
College of Veterinary Medicine
2407 River Drive
Room A-104-C
Knoxville TN 37996-4550

Texas
Texas A & M University
Office of the Dean
College of Veterinary Medicine
& Biomedical Sciences
College Station TX 77843-4461

Virginia
Virginia-Maryland Regional College
of Veterinary Medicine
Admissions Coordinator
Blacksburg VA 24061

Washington
Washington State University
Office of Student Services
College of Veterinary Medicine
100 Grimes Way
P.O. Box 647012
Pullman WA 99164-7012

Wisconsin
University of Wisconsin-Madison
Office of Academic Affairs
School of Veterinary Medicine
2015 Linden Drive
Madison WI 53706-1102

International

Australia
Murdoch University
Murdoch International
South Street
Murdoch 6150
Western Australia

University of Melbourne
Faculty of Veterinary Science
Corner Park Drive and
Flemington Road
Parkville
Melbourne 3010
Victoria Australia

University of Queensland – Gatton
Campus
School of Veterinary Science
Gatton, 4343
Queensland, Australia

University of Sydney
Faculty of Veterinary Science
Sydney, NSW 2006
Australia

School of Veterinary Science
University of Queensland – Gatton
Campus
Gatton, 4343
Queensland, Australia

Canada
Alberta
University of Calgary
Admissions Office
Faculty of Veterinary Medicine
TRW 2D03
3280 Hospital Drive NW
Calgary, AB T2N 4Z6

Montréal
Université de Montréal
Service des Admissions
C.P. 6205
Succursale Centre-Ville
Montréal Québec H3C 3T5 Canada

Ontario
University of Guelph
Admissions Services
University Centre, Level 3
Guelph Ontario N 1G 2W 1
Canada

Prince Edward Island
University of Prince Edward Island
Registrar's Office
Atlantic Veterinary College
550 University Avenue
Charlottetown PEI C1A 4P3
Canada

Saskatchewan
University of Saskatchewan
Admissions Office
Western College of Veterinary
   Medicine
52 Campus Drive
Saskatoon Saskatchewan S7N 5B4
Canada

Caribbean
Ross University School of Veterinary
   Medicine
Office of Admissions
630 US HWY 1
North Brunswick, NJ 08902

St. George's University
Office of Admission
St. George's University
c/o The North American
   Correspondent
University Support Services, LLC
3500 Sunrise Highway
Building 300
Great River, NY 11739

England
Royal Veterinary College
Head of Admissions
Royal College Street
London NW1 0TU
England

Ireland
University College Dublin
Veterinary Medicine Applications
UCD Admissions Office
Tierney Building
Belfield, Dublin 4
Ireland

Mexico
Universidad Nacional Autónoma de
   México
Office of Undergraduate Studies
   (Division de Estudios Profesionales)
College of Veterinary Medicine
   (FMVZ)
Av. Universidad 3000
Circuito Interior
Delegacion Coyoacan
Mexico D.F. 04510

The Netherlands

Utrecht University
Office for International Cooperation
Faculty of Veterinary Medicine
Yalelaan 1
3584 CL Utrecht
The Netherlands

New Zealand

Massey University Veterinary School
International Student Affairs
Undergraduate Office
IVABS
Massey University
Private Bag 11-222
Palmerston North 4442
New Zealand

Scotland

The University of Edinburgh
Admissions Office
Royal (Dick) School of Veterinary
 Studies
Easter Bush Veterinary Centre
Roslin EH25 9RG
Scotland

University of Glasgow
Director of Admissions & Student
 Services Manager
College of Medicine, Veterinary and
 Life Sciences
School of Veterinary Medicine
 Undergraduate School
464 Bearsden Road
Glasgow G61 1QH

Geographical Listing of AAVMC Affiliate (Non-AVMA/COE Accredited) Veterinary Schools and Directory of Admissions Offices

Caribbean

St. Matthew's University
Office of Admissions
12124 High Tech Avenue,
Suite 350
Orlando, Fl 32817

Denmark

University of Copenhagen
Office for International Cooperation
Faculty of Health and Medicine
Blegdamsvej 3B
DK-2200 Copenhagen N
Denmark

LISTING OF CONTRACTING STATES AND PROVINCES

Six Canadian provinces and 19 states in the United States have a veterinary school contract with one or more schools to provide access to veterinary medical education for their residents. The state or province, working through the contracting agency, usually agrees to pay a fee to help cover the cost of education for a certain number of places in each entering class. Residents from the contract states then compete with each other for those positions.

Some states contract with more than one school. For example, Arkansas contracts with 5 veterinary schools, and North Dakota has contracts with 6 schools. Connecticut, Rhode Island, Vermont, Nebraska, and the District of Columbia presently have no contracts, so all candidates from these places apply as nonresidents to veterinary schools of their choice.

The educational agreements between contracting agencies and veterinary schools differ. Under some contract arrangements, students pay in-state tuition; in others, they pay nonresident tuition. Some contract states require students to repay all or part of the subsidy that the state provided; others require veterinary graduates to return to practice in the state for a period of time. Applicants should be aware of their obligation to the state before agreeing to participate in a contract program.

Following is a list of states and provinces that have educational agreements with schools of veterinary medicine.

UNITED STATES

Arizona
Contracts through WICHE* with University of California, Colorado State University, Oregon State University, and Washington State University.

Arkansas
Contracts in past with Louisiana State University, University of Missouri, and Oklahoma State University. Contracts not all completed at time of printing; may be some changes.

Connecticut
Contracts with Iowa State University.

Delaware
Contracts with Oklahoma State University and the University of Georgia.

* WICHE = Western Interstate Commission for Higher Education (offices in Boulder, Colorado)

12

Hawaii
Contracts through WICHE* with University of California, Colorado State University, Oregon State University, and Washington State University.

Idaho
Contracts with Washington State University.

Kentucky
Contracts with Auburn University and Tuskegee University.

Montana
Contracts through WICHE* with University of California, Colorado State University, Oregon State University, and Washington State University.

Nebraska
Formal education alliance with Iowa State University.

Nevada
Contracts through WICHE* with University of California, Colorado State University, Oregon State University, and Washington State University.

New Mexico
Contracts through WICHE* with University of California, Colorado State University, Oregon State University, and Washington State University.

North Dakota
Contracts with Iowa State University, Kansas State University, and the University of Minnesota. Contracts through WICHE* with the University of California, Colorado State University, Oregon State University, and Washington State University.

South Carolina
Contracts with University of Georgia , Mississippi State University, and Tuskegee University.

South Dakota
Reciprocity with University of Minnesota. Contracts with Iowa State University.

Utah
Contracts through WICHE* with University of California, Colorado State University, and Oregon State University. Contracts with Washington State University.

West Virginia
Contracts with Tuskegee University, Mississippi State University, Auburn University, and Virginia-Maryland Regional College of Veterinary Medicine.

Wyoming
Contracts through WICHE* with the University of California, Colorado State University, Oregon State University, and Washington State University.

* WICHE = Western Interstate Commission for Higher Education (offices in Boulder, Colorado)

CANADA

Alberta
Contracts with University of Saskatchewan and University of Calgary.

British Columbia
Contracts with University of Saskatchewan.

Manitoba
Contracts with University of Saskatchewan.

New Brunswick
Contracts with Atlantic Veterinary College at the University of Prince Edward Island and Université de Montréal.

Newfoundland
Contracts with Atlantic Veterinary College at the University of Prince Edward Island.

Nova Scotia
Contracts with Atlantic Veterinary College at the University of Prince Edward Island.

* WICHE = Western Interstate Commission for Higher Education (offices in Boulder, Colorado)

Programs for Multicultural or Disadvantaged Students

The Association of American Veterinary Medical Colleges affirms the value of diversity within the veterinary medical profession. The membership is committed to incorporating that belief into their actions by advocating the recruitment and retention of underrepresented persons as students and faculty and ultimately fostering their success in the profession of veterinary medicine. The Association believes that through these actions society and the profession will be well served.

Many schools have programs designed to facilitate entry into, and retention by, veterinary programs nationwide. These programs are directed at several levels, from high-school students to the student who has already been accepted by a veterinary college. Most of these programs will accept students from every state, regardless of the school(s) to which an individual might eventually apply or attend.

Following is an alphabetical list of schools by state and a short explanation of their programs:

University of California

Program: Summer Enrichment Program

Description: a 6-week summer program. The purpose of this program is to increase the academic preparedness of disadvantaged students through science-based learning skills development, clinical education, individual advising, and student development.

Eligibility: Educationally and/or economically disadvantaged. Must have completed at least one year of college with a minimum science GPA of 2.8 and demonstrated interest in veterinary medicine.

Program dates: July–August.

Contact: Office of the Dean–Student Programs, School of Veterinary Medicine, University of California, One Shields Avenue, Davis CA 95616; telephone: (530) 752-1383.

Sponsorship: School of Veterinary Medicine, University of California-Davis.

Colorado State University

Program: Vet Prep

Description: a one-year academic program that serves as a bridge to the professional veterinary medical program for disadvantaged (cultural, social, eco-

nomic) applicants who ranked high but were denied admission during the current admissions process. Limited to 10 students who upon successful completion are guaranteed admission to the veterinary program. Candidates are selected from the current regular admissions applicant pool.
Eligibility: disadvantaged students.
Contact: College of Veterinary Medicine and Biomedical Sciences, W102 Anatomy, Colorado State University, Fort Collins CO 80523; telephone: (970) 491-7051; email: DVMAdmissions@colostate.edu.
Sponsorship: College of Veterinary Medicine and Biomedical Sciences, Colorado State University.

Program: Vet Start
Description: an 8-year undergraduate and professional program for students who enter Colorado State from high school resulting in a bachelor's and a professional degree. Undergraduate and professional program scholarships are provided, and admission to the professional veterinary medical program is guaranteed upon successful completion of the undergraduate requirements. Mentoring, support services, and summer jobs are available to participants.
Eligibility: students who have a disadvantaged background (economic, cultural, or social) will be given special consideration. Students must be high-school graduates with fewer than 15 semester credits of college coursework post high school graduation. Selection is competitive. There are 5 positions per year for incoming freshman undergraduate students.
Program dates: begins fall semester; applications available online early December; application deadline typically March 1.
Contact: College of Veterinary Medicine and Biomedical Sciences, Campus Delivery 1601, Colorado State University, Fort Collins CO 80523-1601; telephone: (970) 491-7051; email: ken.blehm@colostate.edu.
Sponsorship: College of Veterinary Medicine and Biomedical Sciences, Colorado State University.

Cornell University

Program: State University of New York Graduate Underrepresented Minority Fellowships
Description: all matriculating underrepresented minorities are eligible (not restricted by state residency).
Contact: Director of Student Financial Planning, Office of Student & Academic Services, College of Veterinary Medicine, Cornell University, S2-009 Schurman Hall, Ithaca NY 14853-6401; telephone: (607) 253-3766; www.vet.cornell.edu/financialaid/.

Michigan State University

Program: Vetward Bound Program

Description: Vetward Bound offers different levels of programming, each with its own eligibility requirements. The program provides a review of basic science content, research and/or clinical experience, preparation for the GRE, veterinary experience, food and fiber animal experience, study strategy development, and field experiences. Level placement is determined by program staff and is based on educational background.

Eligibility: Economically and educationally disadvantaged first year undergraduate students through prematriculants into the professional degree program. Students selected to participate will meet HHS Health Careers Opportunity Program guidelines and Federal thresholds. An individual will be determined to be disadvantaged if he or she comes from a background that has inhibited the individual from obtaining the knowledge, skills, and abilities required to enroll in and graduate from a health professions school or comes from a family with an annual income below a level based on low income thresholds according to family size published by the Bureau of the Census, adjusted annually for changes in the Consumer Price Index, and adjusted by the Secretary for use in health professions programs.

Program dates: June–July.

Contact: Vetward Bound Coordinator, College of Veterinary Medicine, 784 Wilson Road, F-110 Veterinary Medical Center, Michigan State University, East Lansing MI 48824; telephone: (517) 355-6521; email: vetbound@cvm. msu.edu.

Mississippi State University

Program: Board of Trustees of State Institutions of Higher Learning Veterinary Medicine Minority Loan/Scholarship Program

Description: a financial assistance program for Mississippi residents who are underrepresented minorities. The loan to service obligation is one year for each year of scholarship assistance, not to exceed four years.

Contact: Susan Eckels, Program Administrator, Mississippi Institutions of Higher Learning, 3825 Ridgewood Road, Jackson MS 39211-6453; telephone: (800) 327-2980.

North Carolina State University

Program: UNC Campus Scholarship Program—Graduate Student Component

Description: UNC General Administration funds this program. Eligibility is limited to new or continuing full-time doctoral students who have financial need and who are residents of North Carolina as of the beginning of the award period (as determined under the *Manual to Assist the Public Higher Education Institutions of N.C. in the Matter of Student Resident Classification for Tuition Purposes).* Individuals who have been accepted to a master's degree program in a department offering the doctoral degree and who intend, and will be eligible, to pursue doctoral studies at NC State after completion of the requirements for the master's degree are also eligible. The program provides up to $3,000 annually for North Carolina residents.

Contact: Director of Diversity Affairs, College of Veterinary Medicine, North Carolina State University, 1060 William Moore Drive, Box 8401, Raleigh, NC 27607; telephone: (919) 513-6262; website: www.cvm.ncsu.edu.

Program: Diversity Graduate Assistant Grant

Description: Funded by the North Carolina State University Graduate School, recipients must be full-time, new or continuing students pursuing master's and doctoral degrees at North Carolina State University. The program provides up to $3,000 annually. Both resident and nonresident students are eligible to apply.

Contact: Director of Diversity Affairs, College of Veterinary Medicine, North Carolina State University, 1060 William Moore Drive, Box 8401, Raleigh, NC 27607; telephone: (919) 513-6262; website: www.cvm.ncsu.edu.

Note: North Carolina residents are encouraged to apply for both programs. However, the annual maximum award for these grant programs is a combined $3,000 (with an option of $500 in additional support for study in the summer). The grant is awarded on an annual basis. Awardees must reapply each year.

The Ohio State University

Program: Young Scholars Program

Description: this summer program is offered to seventh- through eleventh-grade students from Ohio. It provides hands-on science activities, academic enrichment exercises, and career exploration opportunities.

Eligibility: disadvantaged students recommended by their faculty.

Program dates: June to August each summer.

Sponsorship: the State of Ohio and The Ohio State University.

Program: Summer Research Opportunity Program

Description: this program is designed to promote the migration of minority undergraduate students into graduate research educational programs by providing them with summer research experiences. The student is provided with his or her individualized research problem by a faculty mentor and expected to carry that research through to publication.

Eligibility: the student must have completed 2 years of college work and have achieved at least a 2.50 cumulative GPA. The student must be an underrepresented minority or economically disadvantaged.

Contact: Graduate School, The Ohio State University, 230 North Oval Mall, Columbus OH 43210.

Sponsorship: the Big Ten Consortium for Institutional Studies.

18

Purdue University

Program: Access to Animal-Related Careers (A²RC)

Description: A²RC is a two-week, residential program offering hands-on experiences in multiple areas of veterinary medicine including swine production medicine, small animal medicine, and equine medicine. Also included are sessions on several specialty areas such as cardiology, emergency and critical care medicine, and radiology. The program is designed to expose participants to life as a first year DVM student. Mock admissions interviews are conducted and participants are given individual feedback.

Eligibility: A²RC is targeted to 2nd and 3rd year underrepresented minority undergraduate students at partner institutions enrolled in pre-veterinary studies.

Program dates: May 12–25, 2013

For more information on the A²RC program, and to obtain an application, please contact the PVM Director of Diversity Initiatives (contact information below).

Contact: Dr. Kauline Cipriani Davis, Director of Diversity Initiatives (cipriank @purdue.edu or 765 496-1940; website http://www.vet.purdue.edu/diversity/index.php)

University of Tennessee

Program: Veterinary Summer Experience for Tennessee High School Students

Description: The College of Veterinary Medicine offers an eight-week program that provides high school students an opportunity to gain experience working with veterinarians at a veterinary practice in their home towns for seven weeks during the summer. During the eighth week of this summer experience, students will be guests of the College of Veterinary Medicine on the campus of The University of Tennessee in Knoxville. Students will attend clinical rotations in the Equine, Farm Animal, Small Animal, and Avian and Exotic Animal (including zoo medicine) Hospitals in the Veterinary Medical Center. Students will also attend special educational functions related to veterinary medicine.

Eligibility: To qualify for this summer program, a student must be a Tennessee resident and be at least 16 years of age by June 1, be enrolled as a senior or junior in a Tennessee high school, and have earned a minimum 3.0 high school GPA. Applicants must also have an interest in veterinary medicine as a potential career. Preference will be given to applicants who will contribute greatly to the diversity of the summer program and, potentially, to the veterinary profession. Students receive a financial stipend for satisfactory performance in the eight-week program.

Program dates: Summer

Contact: Dr. William Hill, The University of Tennessee, College of Veterinary Medicine, 2431 Joe Johnson Drive, 339 Ellington Plant Science, Knoxville TN 37996, telephone: (865) 974-5770. E-mail: wahill@utk.edu.

University of Minnesota

Program: Veterinary Leadership in Early Admissions for Diversity (VetLEAD)

Description: VetLEAD creates a pathway into the DVM program for high-ability students at under-represented serving partner schools, including Florida Agricultural and Mechanical University (FAMU).

Eligibility: Any high-achieving student enrolled in the Animal Science program at FAMU may apply for an early admissions decision at the end of their sophomore year of undergraduate studies. Eligible students have past experience working or volunteering in a veterinary related setting, a FAMU cumulative GPA of 3.4 with coursework consistent with required prerequisite courses, and strong letters of references.

Contact: Karen Nelson, Director of Admissions, dvminfo@umn.edu

Tuskegee University

Program: Summer Enrichment and Reinforcement Program (SERP) Description: this 6 -week preadmission program is designed to provide academic enrichment through effective learning strategies and mentorship to facilitate the entry of "at risk" students into the veterinary program and successful transition through the professional curriculum .

Description: this 8-week preadmission activity is designed to facilitate the entry of "at risk" students and provide the skills necessary for successful transition to the professional school.

Eligibility: participation is targeted to minority and disadvantaged students who have completed at least 3 years of college and all preveterinary prerequisites. Participation is restricted to persons who have applied to the DVM program in the College of Veterinary Medicine, Nursing, and Allied Health and who have been recommended by the Veterinary Admissions Committee for evaluation to the program.

Program dates: the summer before fall semester.

Contact: Associate Dean for Academic Affairs , College of Veterinary Medicine, Nursing and Allied Health, Tuskegee University, Tuskegee, AL 36088.

Sponsorship: this program is sponsored by a grant from the U.S. Department of Health and Human Services.

Program: Veterinary Science Training, Education and Preparation Institutes for Minority Students (Vet-Step I and II)

Description: Consists of 2 one-week programs designed to encourage high achieving minority students to consider veterinary medicine as a career choice. The program focus on progressive learning skills in reading comprehension, study skills, time-management, note-taking, medical vocabulary, etc.

Eligibility: Vet-Step I accepts 30 students from grades 9 and 10; Vet-Step II accepts students from Vet-Step I and from grade 12. Minority high school honor students interested in the biomedical sciences are strongly encouraged to apply.

Contact: Coordinator, Vet-Step Program, College of Veterinary Medicine, Nursing, and Allied Health, Tuskegee University, Tuskegee AL 36088, (334) 727-8309.

Sponsorship: U.S. Department of Health and Human Services.

Virginia-Maryland Regional College of Veterinary Medicine

Program: Multicultural Academic Opportunities Program

Description: a 10-week program providing opportunities to conduct scientific research; participate in clinical rotations within the veterinary teaching hospital; improve leadership, public speaking, and self-marketing skills; attend GRE preparatory classes; and learn about admission into graduate / professional school.

Contact: Admissions Office at Blacksburg campus.

Program: Summer Research Apprenticeship Program—College Park

Description: a summer research program providing research experience to veterinary and preveterinary students from diverse backgrounds, including economic hardship and underrepresented racial/ethnic groups. Projects may include assisting in the planning, preparation, and data collection for controlled experiments, clinical trials, or epidemiological investigations; researching disease processes; and performing literature searches.

Contact: Admissions Office at College Park campus.

Scholarship Opportunities: a limited number of scholarships are available to assist minority DVM students.

Washington State University

Program: Short-Term Research Training Program for Veterinary Students

Description: a 3-month summer program designed to promote interest in research by veterinary students. Emphasis is on a hands-on research project supervised by a faculty member with a research program. Stipends are provided.

Eligibility: WSU veterinary students or ethnic minority veterinary students from other U.S. colleges of veterinary medicine.

Program dates: 3 months in the summer dependent upon the summer vacation of the WSU College of Veterinary Medicine in which the veterinary student is enrolled.

Contact: Department of Veterinary Microbiology and Pathology, Washington State University, Pullman WA 99164-7040.

Sponsorship: The National Center for Research Resources.

University of Wisconsin

Program: Pre-College Enrollment Opportunity Program for Learning Excellence (PEOPLE)

Description: this program began in the summer of 1999 as a partnership between the Milwaukee Public Schools and the UW-Madison with a group of students who had just completed the ninth grade. New classes will be added each year, expanding to Madison area schools. The program is designed with a precollege track and a bridge program to undergraduate work and continues through a student's undergraduate career at University of Wisconsin-Madison. The main purposes are to promote academic preparation, increase enrollment in postsecondary institutions, and improve retention and graduation rates of minority and disadvantaged students.

Eligibility: students of one or more of the following ethnic heritages: African American, American Indian, Asian American, Hispanic/Latino. Other eligibility factors include economic disadvantage and current enrollment in or commitment to a college preparatory curriculum track.

Program dates: June–July summer residential programs and year-round non-residential programs.

Contact: PEOPLE Program, 1305 Linden Drive, University of Wisconsin- Madison, Madison, WI 53706.

Financial Aid Information

Financing your veterinary medical education requires careful planning, good money management skills, and a willingness to make short-term sacrifices to achieve long-range goals.

Many of you will apply for and receive some type of financial assistance during your undergraduate education. This will help you become somewhat familiar with the process, and to know that the rules and regulations governing programs can and do change periodically.

As a professional student, you will be entering a partnership with the financial aid office, which will require you to complete the appropriate financial aid forms accurately, meet required deadlines, and submit any additional information that may be requested. In return, the financial aid office will determine your aid eligibility and make awards based on the available programs. Your financial aid eligibility takes into account the cost of your education minus any other available resources. Amounts of assistance and the school policies for awarding assistance vary from one veterinary medical school to another and from year to year.

Any questions or concerns that you may have about this topic need to be directed to each of the appropriate financial aid offices to ensure that you receive accurate information and guidance.

Financing Your Veterinary Medical Education

Your education is one of the biggest investments you will make in your lifetime, and one of your most important goals should be to maximize the return on all of your investments. To reach this goal, you must take an active role in managing your financial resources. You need to understand and implement good financial practices. To get you started, here are some good financial habits you should adopt:

- Do not use credit cards to extend your lifestyle. Deciding not to use credit cards except in emergencies is one of the most important decisions you can make, and one that will reduce your stress while you are pursuing your education.
- Budget your money just as carefully as you budget your time. Contact a financial aid administrator to help you set up a budget that will be easy to follow.
- Distinguish between wants and needs. Before you make any purchase, you should ask yourself, "Do I need this, or do I want it?"
- Be a well-informed borrower. If you have not previously taken an active role in understanding the differences between various

student loan programs, now is the time to do it. You need to know these differences in order to avoid high-interest loans and to borrow wisely.

- Borrow the minimum amount necessary in order to maximize the return on your educational investment.
- Be thrifty. Live as cheaply as you can. Remember, you are a student. You'll enjoy a more comfortable lifestyle once you are a DVM.
- Pay any interest that accrues on student loans if you can afford to do so, rather than let the interest accrue and capitalize. Any amount you pay while you're a student will save you money once you enter repayment.

What is the most important piece of advice for making the most of your educational investment? Don't live the lifestyle of a DVM until you have completed your education. Get in the habit of being thrifty. If you live like a DVM while you are in school, you may have to live like a student when you are a DVM.

FEDERAL LOAN PROGRAMS

Please note that subsidized loans are not available beginning fall 2012.

	William D. Ford Unsibsidized Stafford Loan	Perkins Loan	Health professions Student Loan	Loan for Disadvantaged Students	Grad Plus Loans for Graduate/Professional Students
Lender	Federal Loan Program	Federal Loan Program	Federal Loan Program	Federal Loan Program	Federal Loan Program
Financial Need	No	Yes	Yes	Yes	No
Citizenship Requirement	U.S. Citizen, U.S. National or U.S. Permanent Resident	U.S. Citizen, U.S. National or U.S. Permanent Resident	U.S. Citizen, U.S. National or U.S. Permanent Resident	U.S. Citizen, U.S. National or U.S. Permanent Resident	U.S. Citizen, U.S. National or U.S. Permanent Resident
Borrowing Limits	Cost of attendance minus other aid; $189,125 aggregate undergraduate and graduate	$6,000/year; $40,000 aggregate undergraduate and graduate	Cost of attendance at participating school	Federal Loan Programs	Cost of attendance minus other aid
Interest Rate	Fixed; capped at 6.8%	5%	5%	5%	7%
Interest Accrues While Enrolled in School	Yes	No	No	No	Yes
Deferments	Yes	Yes	Yes	Yes	Yes
Grace Period	Yes	Yes	Yes	Yes	No

April 15th Acceptance Deadline Policy

In order to grant member schools enough time to complete their admissions processes and for applicants to make informed admissions decisions, schools will not require applicants to decide upon admissions offers, scholarships and financial aid, until April 15. To ensure applicant awareness of this policy, the schools will attach the policy to all admissions offer letters. If April 15 falls upon a weekend, the date will be shifted to the next Monday.

This policy does not apply to the following schools:
- International Schools
- Tuskegee University

Approved by the AAVMC Board of Directors
July 17, 2011

INFORMATION ABOUT STANDARDIZED TESTS

Most veterinary medical colleges require one or more standardized tests: the Graduate Record Examination (GRE®) or the Medical College Admission Test (MCAT). For further information regarding test dates and registration procedures, contact the testing agencies listed below:

GRE Graduate Record Examinations
P.O. Box 6000
Princeton NJ 08541-6000
(609) 771-7670 (Princeton, N.J.)
also: (510) 654-1200 (Oakland, Calif.)
www.gre.org
Individual school codes: see GRE booklet

MCAT Medical College Admission Test
MCAT Program Office
P.O. Box 4056
Iowa City IA 52243-4056
(319) 337-1357
www.aamc.org/students/mcat/

TOEFL Test of English as a Foreign Language
TOEFL/TSE Services
P.O. Box 6151
Princeton NJ 08541-6151
(609) 771-7100
www.toefl.org

VETERINARY MEDICAL COLLEGE APPLICATION SERVICE (VMCAS)

The Veterinary Medical College Application Service is a centralized application service sponsored by the Association of American Veterinary Medical Colleges. Applicants use VMCAS to apply to most of the AVMA accredited colleges in the United States and abroad.

VMCAS collects, processes, and ships application materials to veterinary colleges designated by the applicant, and responds to applicant inquiries about the application process. This service is the data collection, processing, and distribution component of the admission process for colleges participating in VMCAS. VMCAS, however, does not take part in the admissions selection process.

Twenty-five (25) of the twenty-eight (28) U.S. veterinary institutions participate in VMCAS, along with two (2) Canadian, two (2) Scottish, one (1) English, one (1) Irish, one (1) Australian, and one (1) New Zealand veterinary institutions. Application material deadlines, prerequisite courses, and other aspects of the admissions process differ from school to school. Applicants are responsible for being informed of all instructions provided by VMCAS and the associated member colleges. Questions about using VMCAS should be directed to the VMCAS Student & Advisor Hotline.

Application Cycle Timeline

VMCAS goes live: 1st week in June
VMCAS Application Deadline: Wednesday, October 2, 2013 1:00 PM ET
Transcripts due to VMCAS: September 1, 2013
Fall Transcripts due to VMCAS: February 1, 2013
AAVMC Acceptance Deadline: April 15, 2014
Please be sure to verify individual school deadlines

Key Online Resources

General Information Chart

A one-stop comparison of school info such as location, tuition, seat availability, etc.
http://www.aavmc.org/data/files/vmcas/generalinfo.pdf

Prerequisite Comparison Chart

A course requirement comparison chart of all AAVMC member schools.
http://www.aavmc.org/data/files/vmcas/prerequisites.doc

Test Chart

A showcase of the individual school test requirements and deadlines.
http://aavmc.org/applicant-responsibilities/requirements.aspx (Scroll down to "test scores")

Fee Structure

VMCAS fees broken down by number of designations.
http://aavmc.org/Applicant-Responsibilities/Fees.aspx

Evaluation Requirements

Individual recommendation requirements by school.
http://aavmc.org/Applicant-Responsibilities/Evaluations.aspx

Supplemental Applications

Additional applications required by some schools.
http://www.aavmc.org/supplemental.aspx

Please note that the phone and fax numbers for VMCAS have changed. The mailing address for Transcripts and other VMCAS related correspondences will be changing as of May, 2013, so please go to: http://aavmc.org/vmcas updates.aspx for more critical information.

VMCAS
   1101 Vermont Ave NW
   Suite 301
   Washington, DC 20005
   Telephone (617) 612-2884
   Fax (617) 612-2051
   vmcasinfo@vmcas.org
   http://www.aavmc.org

VETERINARY MEDICAL SCHOOLS IN THE UNITED STATES

AVMA / COE ACCREDITED

Auburn University

Office for Academic Affairs
Auburn University
College of Veterinary Medicine
217 Goodwin/Overton
Auburn AL 36849-5536
Telephone: (334) 844-2685
Email: admiss@vetmed.auburn.edu
www.vetmed.auburn.edu

The College of Veterinary Medicine at Auburn University is located in south central Alabama off Interstate 85 between Montgomery and Atlanta. The university is known for its friendly small-campus atmosphere despite having more than 25,000 students.

Veterinary medicine began as a department at Auburn in 1892 and became a college in 1907. Today it is situated on 280 acres one mile from the main Auburn campus. In addition, the college has a 700-acre research farm five miles from its campus. The college is fully accredited by the American Veterinary Medical Association.

Application Information

For specific application information (availability, deadlines, fees, and VMCAS participation), please refer to the contact information listed above.

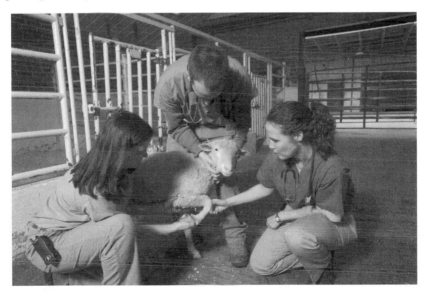

Residency implications: Anticipated class distribution is 40 Alabama residents, 38 Kentucky residents, 2 West Virginia residents and 40 non-contract non-resident students.

Prerequisites for Admission

Course requirements and semester hours

Written composition#	6
* Literature#	3
Fine Arts#	3
Humanities/fine arts elective#	6
* History#	3
Social/behavioral science electives#	9
Mathematics—precalculus with trigonometry#	3
Biology I with lab	4
Biology II with lab	4
Fundamentals of chemistry with lab	8
** Organic chemistry with lab	6
** Physics	8
Biochemistry	3
** Science electives	6
## Animal Nutrition	3

* *Students must complete a 6-semester-hour sequence either in literature or in history.*

** *Organic chemistry, physics, and the two science electives must have been taken within 6 calendar years.*

*** *Science electives must be two of the following: genetics, microbiology, cell biology, comparative anatomy, histology, repro physiology, mammalian or animal physiology, parasitology, embryology, or immunology.*

These requirements will be waived if the student has a bachelor's degree.

Will accept web based or correspondence course.

Required undergraduate GPA: a minimum grade point average of at least 2.50 on a 4.00 scale is required, with the minimum acceptable grade for required courses being C-minus. Applicants not classified as Alabama residents or contract students must have a minimum 3.00 GPA on a 4.00 scale. The mean grade point average of the most recent entering class was 3.53.

AP credit policy: must appear on official college transcripts and be equivalent to the appropriate college-level coursework.

Course completion deadline: prerequisite courses must be completed by June 15 prior to matriculation.

Standardized examinations: Graduate Record Examination (GRE®), general test, is required. The exam must have been taken within the previous 5 calendar years, and must be *received* no later than November 1 of the year of application, therefore you should test no later than October 1st.

Additional requirements and considerations
> Supplemental Application Required - www.vetmed.auburn.edu/admissions
> A minimum of 400 hours of veterinary experience in addition to other animal experience
> Recommendations (3 required)
>> Academic advisor or faculty member
>> Employer
>> Veterinarian
> Extracurricular and community service activities
> Employment record
> Narrative statement of purpose
> Organic chemistry, physics and science electives must have been completed within 6 calendar years

Summary of Admission Procedure

Timetable
> VMCAS application deadline: Wednesday, October 2, 2013 at 1:00 p.m. Eastern Time
> Date interviews are held: February–March
> Date acceptances mailed: March
> School begins: August

Deposit (to hold place in class): none required.

Deferments: not considered.

Transfer Students: Auburn does not take transfer students.

International Students: not considered for admission.

Evaluation criteria
The 3-part admission procedure includes an objective evaluation of academic credentials, a subjective review of personal credentials, and a personal interview by invitation.

2011–2012 admissions summary

	Number of Applicants	Number of New Entrants
Resident	95	40
Contract*	119	40
Nonresident	771	40
Total:	985	120

Expenses for the 2012–2013 Academic Year

Tuition and fees
Resident	$17,440
Nonresident	
Contract*	$17,440
Other nonresident	$41,172

* For further information, see the listing of contracting states and provinces.

Entrance Requirements

Admitted student are residents of Alabama, resident of Kentucky or West Virginia admitted by contract through the Southern Regional Education Board (SREB); or at-large residents (non-Alabama and Non-contract students.) Kentucky students must verify their residency status with their Kentucky pre-vet advisor before October 1. They may contact the Kentucky Council on Postsecondary Education for additional information. West Virginia applicants should verify their residency by contacting Dr. Matthew E. Wilson, Division of Animal & Nutritional Sciences at West Virginia University at (304) 293-3631, extension 4220 or by e-mail at grigs@wvu.edu before October 31.

Resident/contract applicants must be a documented resident of Alabama, Kentucky, or West Virginia and have a minimum grade point average of 2.50 on a 4.0 scale.

University of California

School of Veterinary Medicine
Office of the Dean—Student Programs
University of California
One Shields Avenue
Davis CA 95616
Telephone: (530) 752-1383
www.vetmed.ucdavis.edu

The University of California, Davis (UC Davis) campus is one of 10 campuses of the University of California. It is the largest campus, with 5,200 acres. The Davis campus is set between the Coast Range to the west and the towering Sierra Nevada to the east in the heart of the Central Valley. The campus is close to California's state capital and the San Francisco Bay Area but cherishes its small-town culture and security. Davis is surrounded by open space, including some of the most productive agricultural land in the state. The terrain is flat, and 50 miles of bike paths crisscross the city. Davis has earned the title "City of Bicycles." Winters in Davis are generally mild. Summers are hot and dry, usually in the low 90s, although some days it can exceed 100 degrees. Spring and fall weather is some of the most pleasant in the state. UC Davis is an outstanding research and training institution with over 32,000 undergraduate, graduate and professional students. The Davis campus has four undergraduate colleges, graduate studies in all schools and colleges, and professional programs carried out in the schools of Education, Law, Management, Medicine, Nursing, and Veterinary Medicine. The School of Veterinary Medicine is home of the William R. Pritchard Veterinary Medical Teaching Hospital, Veterinary Medicine Teaching and Research Center, California Animal Health and Food Safety Laboratory, UC Veterinary Medical Center-San Diego, Center for Companion Animal Health and Center for Equine Health. There are many other centers and innovative programs at UC Davis. The school is fully committed to recruiting students with diverse backgrounds.

Application Information

For specific application information (availability, deadlines, fees, and VMCAS participation), please refer to the contact information listed above.

Residency implications: A non-specified number of resident, nonresident, and WICHE applicants are accepted. International students are also considered for admission.

Prerequisites for Admission

Course requirements and quarter hours

General chemistry (with laboratory)	15
Organic chemistry (with laboratory)	6
Physics	6
General biology (with laboratory)	14
Systemic physiology*	5
Biochemistry* (bioenergetics and metabolism)	5
Genetics*	4
English composition and additional English	12
Humanities and social sciences	12
Statistics	4

* Upper-division courses equivalent to one semester or one quarter—labs not required.
Note: equivalent courses may vary in units and may also require other prerequisites. All lower division courses are full year courses on the semester system.

Required undergraduate GPA: a minimum grade point average of 2.50 on a 4.00 scale is required for all science courses completed and 2.50 on all courses cumulatively at time of application. Applicants admitted in fall 2012 had a mean cumulative GPA of 3.63.

AP credit policy: credit and subject title must appear on official college transcripts.

Course completion deadline: all prerequisite courses must be completed by the end of the spring term prior to matriculation. Three-quarters of the required courses must be completed at the time of application.

Standardized examinations: Graduate Record Examination (GRE®), general test is required. The acceptable GRE test dates for applicants entering fall 2013 are September 30, 2008-September 30, 2013. The average GRE scores for the class admitted in 2012 are verbal 574, quantitative 701 and analytical writing 4.55. Only the quantitative score of the GRE will be used as part of the evaluation of the application. All GRE scores must be received by October 15.

Additional requirements and considerations

> Veterinary/animal experience
>> Minimum 180 hrs. of veterinary experience at time of application.
>
> Letters of evaluation (3) and (3) ETS Personal Potential Index (PPI)
>> Evaluations including at least one (1) from a veterinarian. PPI evaluations and VMCAS Letters of evaluation may come from the same people.
>
> Personal statement of motivation/career goals
> Accuracy and neatness of application
> Interview

Summary of Admission Procedure

Timetable
> VMCAS application deadline: Wednesday, October 2, 2013 10:00 a.m.
>> Pacific Standard Time
> No supplemental application required.
> Date interviews are held: mid-December
> Date notifications available via portal: mid-January
> School begins: August

Deposit (to hold place in class): none required.

Deferments: only on case by case basis.

Evaluation criteria
> Grades - Science GPA and Last 45 units
> GRE Quantitative scores
> PPI Evaluations
> MMI Interview

2011–2012 admissions summary

	Number of Applicants	Number of New Entrants
Resident	587	121
Contract*	67	4
Nonresident	488	13
Total:	1,142	138

Expenses for the 2012–2013 Academic Year

Tuition and fees
Resident	$33,091
Nonresident	$45,336
Contract student*	$45,336

* For further information, see the listing of contracting states and provinces. Contract students are not eligible for WICHE funding but all contract and nonresidents may be able to establish residency in California after one year.

Dual-Degree Programs

Combined DVM–graduate degree programs are available.
Visit our Veterinary Scientist Training Program information at
www.vetmed.ucdavis.edu/vstp.

Colorado State University

Colorado State University
College of Veterinary Medicine and Biomedical Sciences
1601 Campus Delivery – Office of the Dean
Fort Collins CO 80523-1601
Telephone: 970-491-7051 or 970-491-7052

Website: http://csu-cvmbs.colostate.edu/dvm-program/Pages/DVM-Program-Entrance-Requirements.aspx

Supplemental Application: http://csu-cvmbs.colostate.edu/dvm-program/Pages/DVM-Application-Procedures.aspx

Email: Students who are enrolled or who plan to be taking lower division courses at CSU prior to admission into the DVM Program, please contact the CSU preveterinary adviser Ann Bowen at ann.bowen@colostate.edu.

Students who are in the planning process of applying to the DVM Program and who are not enrolled in courses at CSU, please email DVMAdmissions@colostate.edu.

Colorado State University is located in Fort Collins, a city of about 150,000 in the eastern foothills of the Rocky Mountains about 65 miles north of Denver. Fort Collins has a pleasant climate and offers many cultural and recreational activities. Many of the state's ski areas lie within a short driving distance, making some of the best skiing in the world accessible. The nearby river canyons and mountain parks are beautiful scenic attractions and provide opportunities for hiking, fishing, photography, camping, and biking.

The College of Veterinary Medicine and Biomedical Sciences is nationally renowned for its programs in oncology, equine surgery and reproduction, and pain management. Our college is composed of eight major buildings that house the departments of biomedical sciences, environmental and radiological health sciences, and microbiology, immunology, and pathology.

The James L. Voss Veterinary Teaching Hospital, one of the world's largest and best-equipped, houses the clinical sciences department. This department boasts a variety of unique units, including the internationally acclaimed Robert H. and Mary G. Flint Animal Cancer Center, Animal Population Health Institute, Integrated Livestock Management Program, and Gail Holmes Equine Orthopaedic Research Center. The hospital attracts a large caseload and offers students a wide variety of clinical experiences.

The uniquely designed Diagnostic Medicine Center houses the college's Veterinary Diagnostic Laboratory (VDL), the university's Extension veterinarian, the Clinical Pathology Laboratory and the Animal Population Health

Institute. The VDL provides disease testing services to veterinarians, state/ federal agencies, livestock owners and pet owners. The Clinical Pathology Laboratory provides services such as blood, fluid and urine analysis and cytology to identify diseases and illnesses in animals brought to the VTH or to veterinarians in the region. The Animal Population Health Institute encourages collaboration and information and expertise exchange in veterinary epidemiology among scientists at CSU, collaborating institutions and government agencies throughout the world.

Internationally known for its innovative curriculum, our veterinary program provides students with a four-year course of study in veterinary medicine leading to the Doctor of Veterinary Medicine degree. The first two years are conducted on the main campus and include comprehensive coverage of veterinary and biomedical sciences along with integrated hands-on and clinical experiences. During the second two years, students participate in animal care at the Veterinary Teaching Hospital through a series of specialty rotations. Students participate as team members in evaluating patients, meeting with clients, developing treatment plans, and providing hands-on care, all under the supervision of faculty clinicians.

Application Information

Application requirements: The Colorado Supplemental Application is required. For your application to be reviewed by the DVM Admissions Committee, we must receive the following items before the deadline:
- VMCAS Application and Fee
- Colorado Supplemental Application and Fee
- GRE Verbal and Quantitative (self-reported/unofficial) scores

If we do not receive these items before the deadline, your application will be designated as Ineligible. For specific requirements, please refer to the website listed above.

Residency implications: Positions are allocated in three pools as Colorado 75, WICHE contracts 30-35 (Arizona, Hawaii, Montana, Nevada, New Mexico, North Dakota, Wyoming), and Nonsponsored 30-35. Our class size is 138. WICHE students must be certified by their states. Nonsponsored students can be from any state or country.

Prerequisites for Admission

Course requirements and semester hours

Laboratory associated with a biology course	1
Genetics	3
Laboratory associated with a chemistry course	1
Biochemistry	3

Physics (with laboratory)	4
Statistics/biostatistics	3
English composition	3
Social sciences and humanities	12
Electives	30

Required undergraduate GPA: No minimum requirement. The mean GPA for the 2012 matriculated class was 3.60 on a 4.00 scale.

AP credit policy: Must appear on official college transcripts.

Course completion deadline: transcripts with final grades, including all required courses, must be received by July 15 prior to matriculation.

Standardized examinations: The GRE® General Test (Verbal and Quantitative) is required. The mean GRE scores for the 2012 matriculated class are Verbal 537 and Quantitative 664. Test scores dated earlier than October 1, 2008, will not be accepted. It is the *applicant's* responsibility to schedule the test on or before Sept. 27 so s/he can self-report unofficial scores on the Colorado Supplemental Application before the October 2, 2013 11:00am MT deadline. You will know your unofficial scores before leaving the testing center. *NOTE: The self-reported unofficial Verbal and Quantitative scores must be entered into the application in order to submit your application.*

Sending official scores: Applicants should submit a request to their testing center, before Oct. 2, to have official scores sent to CSU. (GRE® code 4075, Dept code 0617). Scores should be received by Nov. 30. In December, *official* scores will be used to verify all applicant *self-reported* scores before offers are made.

Letter of Reference: All applicants will need to request three recommenders to submit a VMCAS electronic letter of recommendation (VMCAS e-LOR) AND an ETS PPI web-based evaluation (for inclusion in the ETS PPI Evaluation Report). BOTH the VMCAS e-LORs AND the ETS PPI Evaluation Report are required; therefore, applicants should ask their recommenders to write and submit the VMCAS e-LOR and the ETS PPI online evaluation. For specific information, please see item #4 at http://csu-cvmbs.colostate.edu/dvm-program/Pages/DVM-Application-Procedures.aspx.

In fairness to all applicants, the Admissions Committee will review no more than three LOR's. CSU suggests one should be from an advisor/professor, one from an employer, and at least one from a veterinarian.

Additional requirements and considerations: Please see "Evaluation Criteria" in the next section.

Summary of Admission Procedure

Timetable
> Colorado Supplemental Application deadline: Wednesday, October 2, 2013 at 11:00 am (MT).
> VMCAS Application deadline: Wednesday, October 2, 2013 at 1:00 p.m. (ET).
> School begins: late August

Deposit (to hold place in class): none required.

Deferments: not considered.

Evaluation criteria
> Quality of academic program (course load, challenging curriculum, honors)
> GRE scores
> Veterinary/animal/ other work experience
> Extracurricular/community activities, achievements, leadership
> Essay
> Contribution to diversity, unique attributes, extenuating circumstances
> Letters of Reference

2012–2013 admissions summary

	Number of Applicants	Number of New Entrants
Sponsored (Colorado)	264	75
Sponsored (WICHE)*	151	36
Nonsponsored	1,079	27
Total:	1,494	138

Estimated expenses for the 2012–2013 Academic Year

Tuition and fees (estimate)
Sponsored (Colorado & WICHE)	$25,242
Nonsponsored	$53,218

* For further information, see the listing of contracting states and provinces.

Dual-Degree Programs

The CVMBS offers combined 5-year MBA/DVM (business), MPH/DVM (public health), and international MST/DVM (toxicology) programs. In addition, we offer a combined 7 8 year DVM/PhD program
http://csu-cvmbs.colostate.edu/dvm-program/Pages/DVM-MBA.aspx
http://csu-cvmbs.colostate.edu/dvm-program/Pages/DVM-MPH.aspx
http://csu-cvmbs.colostate.edu/dvm-program/Pages/DVM-MST.aspx
http://csu-cvmbs.colostate.edu/dvm-program/Pages/DVM-PhD.aspx

Cornell University

Office of Student & Academic Services
College of Veterinary Medicine
S2-009 Schurman Hall
Cornell University
Ithaca, NY 14853-6401
Telephone: (607) 253-3700
Email: vet_admissions@cornell.edu
www.vet.cornell.edu/admissions

Cornell is located in Ithaca, a college town of about 30,000 in the Finger Lakes region of upstate New York, a beautiful area of rolling hills, deep valleys, scenic

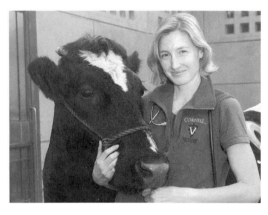

gorges, and clear lakes. The university's 740-acre campus is bounded on two sides by gorges and waterfalls. Open countryside, state parks, and year-round opportunities for outdoor recreation, including excellent sailing, swimming, skiing, hiking, and other activities, are only minutes away.

Ithaca is one hour by air and a four-hour drive from New York City, and other major metropolitan areas are easily accessible. Direct commercial flights connect Ithaca with New York, Boston, Chicago, Pittsburgh, Philadelphia, and other cities.

The tradition of academic excellence, the cultural vigor of a distinguished university, and the magnificent setting create a stimulating environment for graduate study. The curriculum differs from other programs in that it is interdisciplinary, small group learning early in the program and focuses on the student as the primary force in learning.

Application Information

For specific information about the application process visit our web site at http://www.vet.cornell.edu/admissions/. The Supplemental Application can be found at http://www.vet.cornell.edu/admissions/CornellSupplementalApplication.cfm. You may also subscribe to our free electronic Pre-Vet Newsletter at http://www.vet.cornell.edu/admissions/PreVetNewsletters.cfm for application updates and current information about the College of Veterinary Medicine.

Residency implications: approximately 55 seats for New York State residents and 47 seats for non-NY residents.

Prerequisites for Admission

Course requirements and semester hours

English composition/literature* (full year)	6
Biology or zoology, full year with laboratory	6

* Three credits of literature may be satisfied by a course in public speaking.

Physics, full year with laboratory	6
Inorganic (general) chemistry, full year with laboratory	6
Organic chemistry, full year with laboratory	6
Biochemistry, half year required; full year preferred	4
General microbiology, with laboratory	3
Non-prerequisite elective credits needed	53

All prerequisites must have a letter grade of C– or better.

Required undergraduate GPA: No specific GPA requirement, but the grade range of those admitted tends to be 3.00–4.00.

AP credit policy: accepted for physics and general or inorganic chemistry with a score of 4 or higher.

Course completion deadline: all but 12 credits of the prerequisite coursework should be completed at the time of application, with at least one semester of any two-semester series underway. Any outstanding prerequisites must be completed by the end of the spring term prior to matriculation.

Standardized examinations: Graduate Record Examination (GRE®), general test (verbal and quantitative), or the Medical College Admission Test (MCAT) is required. Official test scores must be received directly from ETS or AMA by Oct. 15. (Last recommended date to take tests is September 30.) Test scores older than 5 years will not be accepted.

Additional requirements and considerations

- Up to 5 most significant animal/veterinary/biomedical research experiences listed on the Cornell Supplemental Application with letters of evaluation (evaluations can come through the eLor system or the Cornell electronic evaluation system
- At least one letter of evaluation from a veterinarian
- Academic advisor or faculty evaluation
- Extracurricular and/or community service activities; Non-veterinary work experiences
- Essay and short answer questions

Summary of Admission Procedure

Timetable
> VMCAS application deadline: Wednesday, October 2, 2013 at 1:00 p.m.
>   Eastern Time (transcripts due September 1, 2013, to VMCAS)
> Supplemental application deadline: Oct. 15
> Information sessions at the college for admitted students and
>   alternates: February/March
> Date acceptances mailed: January
> School begins: mid/late August

Deposit (to hold place in class): $500.00 (by April 15).

Deferments: considered on an individual basis, and ordinarily granted for illness or other situations beyond the control of the applicant.

Evaluation criteria
The following admissions formula allows the applicant to see how their application will be reviewed:

> 25% Overall GPA
> 25% GRE (verbal & quantitative) or MCAT Scores
> 20% Animal/Veterinary/Biomedical Research Experiences
>   • at least one letter of evaluation from a veterinarian
> 5% Quality of Academic Program
>   • with academic letter of evaluation
> 10% Non-Cognitive Skills
> 10% All Other Achievements
> 5% Personal Statement

2011–2012 admissions summary

	Number of Applicants	Number of New Entrants
Resident	261	54
Nonresident*	656	48
Total:	917	102

* All other states and international applicants.

Expenses for the 2012–2013 Academic Year

Tuition and fees

Resident	$29,400
Nonresident	$44,250

Dual-Degree Programs

DVM/PhD Dual Degree- By integrating Cornell's veterinary and graduate curricula in the DVM/PhD Program, we prepare students to become leaders in science, medicine, and society, able to excel in basic research, cutting-edge medicine, and teaching. Students receive substantial financial funding incentives to complete both degrees.

DVM/MPH (Masters in Public Health)- A partnership between the College of Veterinary and the University of Minnesota School of Public Health allows students the opportunity to earn a Master of Public Health (MPH) degree while completing their DVM training.

For more information on both dual degree programs visit http://www.vet. cornell.edu/admissions/OADualDegree.cfm

Other Admissions Programs

Sophomore Early Acceptance Program- The *Early Acceptance Program* gives exceptionally well qualified applicants the opportunity to obtain admission to veterinary school after the completion of the sophomore year. With admission to the Cornell University College of Veterinary Medicine secured, the successful applicant may use the time between acceptance and matriculation to pursue experience in areas of personal interest. More information can be found at http://www.vet.cornell.edu/admissions/OAEarlyAcceptance.cfm.

Transfer Student Admissions- Cornell will consider applications for advanced standing in the DVM program on an individual basis, if an opening exists in the second-year class. More information can be found at http://www. vet.cornell.edu/admissions/transferstudents.cfm.

Summer Research Opportunities

The Leadership Program for Veterinary Scholars- A unique summer learning experience for veterinary students who seek to broadly influence the veterinary profession through a career in research. The program in an intensive research-oriented learning experience that combines faculty-guided research with career counseling, student-directed learning, and a variety of professional enrichment activities.

Additional Summer Research Opportunities- Additional summer research opportunities for veterinary students include the Veterinary Investigator Program, Veterinary Training in Biomedical Research, Aquavet, Summer Dairy Institute, the Food Animal Medicine Externship, and the Havemeyer Foundation Equine Research Fellowships.

For more information about all of these summer research opportunities visit http://www.vet.cornell.edu/BBS/Scientists/SummerResearch.cfm.

University of Florida

Admissions Office
College of Veterinary Medicine
P.O. Box 100125
University of Florida
Gainesville FL 32610-0125
Telephone: 352-294-4244
Email: chaparrol@ufl.edu
www.vetmed.ufl.edu

The University of Florida is located in Gainesville, a college town of approximately 125,000 in north central Florida, midway between the Gulf of Mexico and the Atlantic Ocean. Changes in season are marked, but winters are mild and permit year-round participation in outdoor activities.

The university accommodates about 50,000+ students with programs in almost all disciplines. The College of Veterinary Medicine is a component of the Institute of Food and Agricultural Sciences (which also includes Agriculture and Forest Resources and Conservation). It is also one of 6 colleges affiliated with the Health Science Center (the other 5 are Dentistry, Public Health and Health Professions, Medicine, Nursing, and Pharmacy).

The veterinary curriculum is a 9-semester program consisting of core curriculum and elective experiences. The core provides the body of knowledge and skills common to all veterinarians. The first 4 semesters concentrate primarily on basic medical sciences. Students are additionally introduced to physical diagnosis, radiology, and clinical problems during these years. The core also includes experience in each of the clinical areas. Elective areas of concentration permit students to investigate further the aspects of both basic and clinical sciences most relevant to their interests.

Application Information

For specific application information (availability, deadlines, fees, and VMCAS participation), please refer to the contact information listed above.

Residency implications: Florida has no contractual agreements. The college admits 88 Florida residents and 24 non-sponsored applicants each academic year. International applicants are included in the non-sponsored pool.

Prerequisites for Admission (subject to change)

Course requirements and semester hours

Biology (general, genetics, microbiology)	15
Chemistry (inorganic, organic, biochemistry)	19

Physics	8
Mathematics (calculus, statistics)	6
Animal Science (introduction to animal science, animal nutrition)	6
Humanities	9
Social sciences	6
English (2 courses in English composition)	6
Electives	at least 5

All pre-requisites must be completed with a grade letter of C or above. Pre-requisites with a letter grade of C- or below must be retaken.

Suggested undergraduate GPA: a minimum GPA of 3.0 on a 4.00 scale. The class of 2016 had an overall mean science prerequisite GPA of 3.47.

AP credit policy: must appear on official college transcripts and be equivalent to the appropriate college-level coursework.

Course completion deadline: prerequisite courses must be completed by the end of the spring term prior to admission.

Standardized examinations: Graduate Record Examination (GRE®) is required. To be considered for Class of 2018 admissions cycle, the last day to seat for the GRE is August 30, 2013. Scores must be received in our office by September 9, 2013. GRE code for our college is 5753. Mean score for the class of 2016 was 1223

Additional requirements and considerations
>   Animal/veterinary experience - at least 500 hours suggested
>   Recommendations/evaluations (3 required)
>>   Veterinarian - two references suggested
>>   Academic advisor/Personal - one reference suggested
>   Honors and awards received
>   Extracurricular activities

Summary of Admission Procedure

Timetable
>   VMCAS application deadline: Wednesday, October 2, 2013 at 1:00 p.m. Eastern Time.
>   UF Professional School Application deadline: September 9, 2013. Information on our supplemental requirements can be found at: www.vetmed.ufl.edu. Note: The University of Florida School of Veterinary Medicine requires three supplemental forms which will be available after completing the UF Professional School Application.

47

Date interviews are held: February
Date acceptances mailed: March
School begins: mid-August

Deposit (to hold place in class): none required.

Deferments: considered on an individual basis.

Evaluation criteria
The admission procedure consists of 3 parts: each applicant's file is reviewed; selected applicants are each interviewed for about 1 hour by 3 admissions committee members; final selection of new class takes place.

2011–2012 admissions summary

	Number of Applicants	Number of New Entrants
Resident	275	88
Contract	N/A	N/A
Nonresident	<u>473</u>	<u>23</u>
Total:	748	111

Expenses for the 2012–2013 Academic Year

Tuition and fees
Resident	$28,100
Non-Sponsored	$45,500

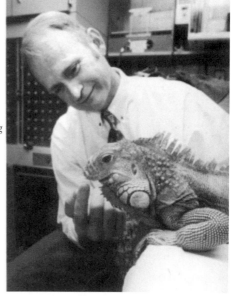

Not all of a veterinarian's patients are cuddly, especially for those specializing in wildlife and zoo medicine. Photo courtesy of University of Florida.

University of Georgia

Admissions Department
Office for Academic Affairs
College of Veterinary Medicine
The University of Georgia
Athens GA 30602-7372
Telephone: (706) 542-5728
www.vet.uga.edu/admissions
email: dvmadmit@uga.edu

The University of Georgia is located in Athens-Clarke County, with a population of over 100,000. Georgia's "Classic City" is a prospering community that reflects the charm of the Old South while growing in culture and industry (www. visitathensga.com). Athens is just over an hour away from the north Georgia mountains and the metropolitan area of Atlanta, and just over 5 hours away from the Atlantic coast.

In 1785, Georgia became the first state to grant a charter for a state-supported university. In 1801 the first students came to the newly formed frontier town of Athens. The University of Georgia has grown into an institution with 16 schools and colleges and more than 2,889 faculty members and 34,519 students.

Application Information

For specific application information (availability, deadlines, fees, and VMCAS participation), please refer to the contact information listed above.

Residency implications: Georgia retains up to 18 positions for contract students. Contracts are with Delaware (maximum 1) and South Carolina (maximum 17). The balance of those admitted are residents of Georgia or nonresident, non-contract applicants. International applications are accepted. Total number of students admitted each year: 102.

Prerequisites for Admission

Course requirements and semester hours

English (writing intensive)	6
Humanities and social studies	14
General biology with lab (for science majors)	8
Advanced biological science*	8
Chemistry with lab	
Inorganic	8
Organic	8

| Physics with lab | 8 |
| Biochemistry (lab not required) | 3 |

*300/3000 level or higher biology courses that have general biology as a prerequisite. Nutrition, behavior and ecology courses typically do not count towards the advanced biological sciences requirement

Required undergraduate GPA: cumulative GPA of 3.00 or greater on a 4.00 scale or a combined score on the GRE® verbal and quantitative sections of 1200 on the old scale or 308 or higher on the new scale.

AP credit policy: must appear on official college transcripts and be equivalent to the appropriate college-level coursework.

Course completion deadline: prerequisite courses must be completed by the end of the spring term preceding entry.

Standardized examinations: Graduate Record Examination (GRE®) general test (including the analytical writing test) must be completed within the 5 years immediately preceding the deadline for receipt of applications (October 2, 2013 at 1:00 p.m. Eastern Time). Test scores must be received electronically from ETS by October 2, 2013 (please consider processing time when requesting your scores to be sent).

Veterinary experience requirement: Applicants must have a minimum of 250 hours of veterinary experience to be considered. To count towards veterinary experience you must be under the direct supervision of a veterinarian. If you are not under the direct supervision of a veterinarian, the experience is considered animal experience.

Additional requirements and considerations
> Supplemental application (available at www.vet.uga.edu)
> Minimum of 250 veterinary experience hours
> Animal experience
> Personal statement
> Background for veterinary medicine
> Electronic Recommendations/evaluations (3 required): Veterinarian
> (required)
>> Academic advisor/faculty member (required for graduate students)
>> Employer

Summary of Admission Procedure

Timetable
> VMCAS application deadline: Wednesday, October 2, 2013 at 1:00 p.m.
> Eastern Time

Supplemental application deadline: October 2, 2013 at 1:00 p.m.
Eastern Time (The deadline to request a supplemental application
account will be posted on our website)
GRE score deadline: October 2, 2013 (scores must be submitted
electronically from ETS)
Date acceptances mailed: mid-March
School begins: mid-August. A required 6-day orientation will precede
the start of classes.

Deposit (to hold place in class): $500; $750 for nonresident, noncontract students.

Deferments: one-year deferments considered on a case-by-case basis.

Evaluation criteria
The admissions procedure includes a file evaluation. There are no interviews.
Program of study
Animal/veterinary experience
References
Employment history
Personal statement
Extracurricular activities

2011–2012 admissions summary

	Number of Applicants	Number Accepted
Resident	218	73
Contract*	66	18
Nonresident	426	11
Total:	710	102

Expenses for the 2012–2013 Academic Year

Tuition and fees (approximate)
Resident	$17,078
Nonresident	
Contract*	$25,800
Nonresident	$42,878

Dual-Degree Programs

Combined DVM-graduate degree programs are available: DVM-MPH
Veterinarians in Public Health
DVM/PhD Veterinary Medical Scientist Training Program

University of Illinois

University of Illinois
College of Veterinary Medicine
Office of Academic and Student Affairs
2001 South Lincoln Ave., Room 2271G
Urbana IL 61802
Telephone: (217) 265-0380
Email: admissions@vetmed.illinois.edu

The University of Illinois is in Urbana-Champaign, a community of about 100,000 people located 140 miles south of Chicago. It is served by two airlines, 3 interstate highways, bus, and rail. The twin cities and university make a pleasant community with easy access to all areas and facilities. The university has about 42,000 students and more than 11,000 faculty and staff members. It is known for its high-quality academic programs and its exceptional resources and facilities. The university library has the largest collection of any public university and ranks third among all U.S. academic libraries. The university also has outstanding cultural and sports facilities and activities.

The College of Veterinary Medicine is located at the south edge of the campus. In addition to approximately 480 students, the college has about 100 graduate students plus a full complement of residents and interns. There are more than 100 full-time faculty with research interests in a variety of biomedical sciences and clinical areas. This research activity offers a broad variety of experiences for students. The college also offers students a dynamic, integrated core-elective curriculum to prepare for careers in almost any area of the profession.

Application Information

For specific application information (availability, deadlines, fees, and VMCAS participation), please refer to the contact information listed above.

A Supplemental Application specific to the University of Illinois is required and may be obtained from the College Admissions website at: https://vetmed.illinois.edu/admissions/

International applications are considered, although there obvious constraints regarding translation of grades. The TOEFL will be required of any successful applicant before matriculation. U.S. Visa constraints may also be restrictive for admission.

Residency implications: priority is given to approximately 85 Illinois residents; approximately 35 nonresident positions are available.

Prerequisites for Admission

The academic requirements for application to the College of Veterinary Medicine can be met through one of two pathways: Plan A or Plan B. Those considering a career in veterinary medicine should have a good foundation in biological sciences and chemistry, including biochemistry, and should consider the specific courses listed in Plan A as the very minimum knowledge base for success in the curriculum.

Plan A

BS or BA degree in any major field of study from a regionally accredited college or university including the following courses (equivalent in content to those required for students majoring in biological sciences):

- a. 8 semester hours of biological sciences with laboratories
- b. 16 semester hours of chemical sciences, including organic, inorganic and biochemistry, with laboratories in inorganic and organic chemistry
- c. 8 semester hours of physics with laboratories

Plan B

Those applying without a bachelor's degree are required to present at least 60 semester hours from a regionally accredited college or university, including 44 hours of science courses. The minimum course requirements under Plan B are:

- a. 8 semester hours of biological sciences with laboratories
- b. 16 semester hours of chemical sciences, including organic, inorganic and biochemistry, with laboratories in inorganic and organic chemistry
- c. 8 semester hours of physics with laboratories
- d. 3 semester hours of English composition and an additional 3 hours of English composition and/or speech communication
- e. 12 semester hours of humanities and/or social sciences
- f. 12 semester hours of junior/senior-level science courses in addition to the requirements listed above

Applicants must have no more than 2 prerequisite courses to complete following the fall term in which they submit their application. All prerequisites must be complete by the end of the Spring 2014 term.

Required undergraduate GPA: a minimum cumulative GPA of 2.75 and a minimum science GPA of 2.75 on a 4.00 scale are required. The average statistics for students making it past Admissions Phase I in 2012 were 3.59 cumulative GPA, 3.49 science GPA, and 63% GRE composite percentile

AP credit policy: AP credit is allowed to meet the 8 s.h. physics prerequisite requirement if a student is awarded the full 8 s.h. AP credit is allowed for biology and chemistry if it is followed up by more advanced college-level courses in those science areas for physics.

Standardized examinations: Graduate Record Examination (GRE®), general test, is required. Test must be taken by September 15, 2013 for the 2013/2014 admission cycle (no test taken after September 15, 2013 will be considered), and scores may be no older than two years (i.e. August 1, 2011-September 15, 2013). All 3 components of the exam must be completed as one exam. The higher composite score of the two most recent examinations will be used.

Additional requirements and considerations
> Animal and veterinary knowledge, motivation, and experience
> Recommendation/evaluation/suggestions: No more than 5 letters of recommendation will be accepted and no less than 3. One letter should be from a college instructor or academic adviser. One letter should be from a veterinarian familiar with the student's potential and motivation. The third letter may be from a second veterinarian or academician or from an individual who can objectively evaluate your potential and motivation.
> Evidence of leadership, initiative, and responsibility
> Rigor of academic preparation

Summary of Admission Procedure

Timetable
> VMCAS application deadline: Wednesday, October 2, 2013 at 1:00 p.m. Eastern Time (noon Central Time)
> Informational program and required interviews: Mid-February
> National application acceptance date: April 15, 2014
> Date acceptances mailed: late February-early March
> School begins: late August

Deposit (to hold place in class): $500 deposit required on acceptance. Please check the Illinois Admissions website for the most current information.

Deferments: considered on an individual basis by the Associate Dean for Academic and Student Affairs.

Evaluation criteria

A 3-part admission procedure is used. An academic evaluation and an application evaluation of veterinary, animal experience and personal qualities are followed by a personal interview.

Academic evaluation:
{
  GRE® test scores
  Science GPA
  Cumulative GPA
  Rigor of academic preparation
}

Nonacademic evaluation:
{
  veterinary-related experience, animal-related
    experience, community involvement,
    leadership, citizenship, and letters of
    recommendation
}

Interview

2011–2012 admissions summary

	Number of Applicants	Number of New Entrants
Resident	221	97
Nonresident	734	17
Total:	955	114

Expenses for the 2011–2012 Academic Year

Tuition and fees
Resident	$28,446
Nonresident	$44,910

Dual-Degree Programs

Combined DVM/PhD programs may be available. DVM/MPH with concurrent enrollment at University of Illinois at Chicago, School of Public Health are also available.

Iowa State University

Office of Admissions
College of Veterinary Medicine
2270 Veterinary Medicine Iowa State University P.O. Box 3020
Ames IA 50010-3020 Telephone: (515) 294-5337
Toll free outside Iowa: (800) 262-3810
Email: cvmadmissions@iastate.edu
www.vetmed.iastate.edu

The Iowa State University College of Veterinary Medicine is located in the heart of one of the world's most intensive livestock-producing areas, which provides diverse food-animal clinical and diagnostic cases. A nearby metropolitan area and a regionally recognized referral veterinary hospital provide experience in companion-animal medicine and surgery. A strong basic science education during the first 2 years prepares veterinary students for a wide range of clinical experiences during the last 2 years. The College of Veterinary Medicine provides education in a wide variety of animal species and disciplines and allows fourth-year students to spend time with private practitioners, other colleges, research facilities, and in other educational experiences. Opportunities for research exist in the outstanding research programs in neurobiology, immunobiology, infectious diseases, and numerous other areas. The nearby National Animal Disease Center and the National Veterinary Services Laboratories provide additional research opportunities. The world's premier State Diagnostic Laboratory is part of the college and provides students with experience that is unmatched by any other veterinary college in the world. Graduates are highly sought after and can typically choose among 5 or 6 job offers. A career development and placement service is also provided.

Application Information

The most current application information (availability, deadlines, fees, VM-CAS participation), may be found at http://vetmed.iastate.edu/academics/prospective-students/admissions.

Supplemental Application: A supplemental application is required. The supplemental becomes available June 1 and the link can be found at http://vetmed.iastate.edu/academics/prospective-students/admissions.

Residency implications: priority is given to Iowa residents for approximately 60 positions. Iowa contracts on a year-to-year basis with North Dakota, South Dakota and Connecticut. Iowa also has a formal educational alliance with Nebraska. Remaining positions are available for residents of noncontract states or international students.

Prerequisites for Admission

Course requirements and semester hours

English composition[†]	6
General chemistry (1 year series w/lab)	7
Organic chemistry (1 year series w/lab)	7
Biochemistry	3
Physics (Physics 1 – first semester of a two-semester series w/lab)	4
Biology (1 year series w/labs)	8
Genetics (Upper level Mendelian and molecular)	3
Mammalian anatomy and/or physiology	3
Oral communication (interpersonal, group or public speaking)	3
Arts, humanities, or social sciences	8
Electives	8

† English composition of one year or writing emphasis courses (may include business or technical writing). Bachelor's degree fulfills 3 sem cr English composition.

Required undergraduate GPA: the minimum GPA required is 2.50 on a 4.00 scale. The most recent entering class had a mean GPA of 3.55.

AP credit policy: must be documented by original scores submitted to the university, and must meet the university's minimum requirement in the appropriate subject area. CLEP (College-Level Examination Program) credits accepted only for the arts, humanities, and social sciences.

Course completion deadline: It is preferred that prerequisite science courses be completed by the end of the fall term the year the applicant applies, and these must be completed with a C (2.0) or better to fulfill the requirement. However, up to 2 prerequisite science courses may be taken the spring term prior to matriculation. All other prerequisites must be completed by the end of the spring term prior to matriculation with a C (2.0) or better. Pending courses may not be completed the summer prior to matriculation. Pass–not pass grades are not acceptable.

Standardized examinations: Graduate Record Examination (GRE®), general test, is required. Either the new Revised GRE or the previous GRE will be accepted but the scores must come directly from GRE. The last date to take the GRE for Iowa residents is August 15, 2013 and the last date for all other applicants to take the GRE is September 15, 2013. All scores must be received by the listed application deadline date.

Additional requirements and considerations
Recommendations (3 required). Academic advisors, veterinarians, and employers are suggested. The applicant is strongly encouraged to have at least one of these recommendations from a veterinarian. Other suggested evaluators include academic advisors or professors and employers. The evaluator should know the applicant well and be able to speak to their personal characteristics and attributes. It is preferred that the evaluator include comments or a letter with the form evaluation. A letter can be composed in the comments section of the VMCAS electronic letter of recommendation. Evaluators cannot be related to the applicant by blood or marriage.

Letters of recommendation are due the same date and time as the application. Iowa residents: September 3, 2013. All other applicants: October 2, 2013 at 1:00 p.m. Eastern Time. Letters of recommendation sent directly to the ISU-CVM will NOT be accepted. No late letters of evaluation will be allowed.

Summary of Admission Procedure

Timetable
> Application deadline: Iowa Residents: September 3, 2013
> All other applicants: Wednesday, October 2, 2013 at 1:00 p.m.
>   Eastern Time
> Date acceptances mailed: Approximately February 15
> School begins: late August

Deposit (to hold place in class): $500.00.

Deferments: considered on a case-by-case basis.

Evaluation criteria
The admission procedure consists of a review of each candidate's application and qualifications:

1. Academic factors include grades, test scores, and degrees earned.
2. Nonacademic factors include essays, experience, recommendations, and personal development activities.
3. Interviews are conducted.

2011–2012 admissions summary

	Number of Applicants	Number of New Entrants
Resident	131	64
Contract*	155	41
Nonresident	896	44
Total:	1,182	149

Expenses for the 2012–2013 Academic Year

Tuition and fees

Resident	$19,581
Nonresident	
Contract*	varies by contract
Other nonresident	$41,390
Fees (approximate)	$1,077

* For further information, see the listing of contracting states and provinces.

Dual-Degree Programs

Combined DVM–graduate degree programs are available, including a DVM/MPH and DVM/MBA.

Kansas State University

Office of Student Admissions
College of Veterinary Medicine
101 Trotter Hall
Kansas State University
Manhattan KS 66506-5601
Telephone: (785) 532-5660
Fax: (785) 532-5884
Email: admit@vet.k-state.edu
www.vet.k-state.edu

Kansas State University in Manhattan, Kansas, is located 125 miles west of Kansas City near Interstate 70. With a population of about 70,000 including KSU, Manhattan is in an area surrounded by many historical points of interest in a rich agricultural area of north central Kansas. Recreational activities abound in Manhattan and the surrounding area with fishing, boating, camping, and hunting among the favorites. Sporting events, theater, concerts, and excellent parks contribute to the many activities available. Kansans enjoy the 4 seasons, each of which brings its own special activities and events.

Kansas State University is on a beautiful 664-acre campus. The College of Veterinary Medicine opened in 1905. It is located on 80 acres just north of the main campus in 3 connected buildings.

Application Information

For specific application information (availability, deadlines, fees, and VMCAS participation), please refer to the contact information listed above.

Supplemental Application: Available at http://www.vet.k-state.edu/admit/apply. htm between June 1 and October 1

Contract tuition: resident tuition

Resident seats: approximately 45

Contract seats: 5 with North Dakota

Residency implications: to be eligible to be in the Kansas pool of applicants, the applicant must be a Kansas resident for tuition purposes at the time of application. Kansas accepts about 60 nonresident students per year. International applicants are considered. Kansas has a contract for students from North Dakota.

Prerequisites for Admission

Course Requirements and Semester Hours

Expository writing I and II	6
Public speaking	2
Chemistry I and II	8
General organic chemistry, with laboratory	5
General biochemistry	3
Physics I and II	8
Principles of biology or general zoology	4
Microbiology, with laboratory	4
Genetics	3
Social sciences and /or humanities	12
Electives	9

Science courses must have been taken within six years of the date of enrollment in the professional program.

Required undergraduate GPA: the minimum required GPA to qualify for an interview is 2.80 on a 4.00 scale in both the prerequisite courses and the last 45 semester hours of undergraduate work. The most recent entering class had a mean prerequisite science GPA of 3.50.

AP credit policy: must appear on official college transcripts and be equivalent to the appropriate college-level coursework.

Course completion deadline: prerequisite courses must be completed by the end of the spring term of the year in which admission is sought.

Standardized examinations: Graduate Record Examination (GRE®), general test scores are required by October 1, unless all prerequisites are completed at Kansas State University.

Additional requirements and considerations
Animal/veterinary work experience and knowledge
Employment record
3 evaluations required by nonfamily members: one veterinarian, one academic or preprofessional advisor, one professor or other professional.

Summary of Admission Procedure

Timetable
> VMCAS application deadline: Wednesday, October 2, 2013 at 1:00 p.m.
>   Eastern Time
> Kansas State University supplemental application deadline: postmarked
>   by Tuesday, October 1, 2013
> Date interviews are held:
>   Kansas residents: mid-December
>   Nonresident: early January
>   North Dakota: February
> Date acceptances mailed: within 3 weeks after interview
> School begins: mid-August

Deposit (to hold place in class): $500.00.

Deferments: may be considered by Admissions Committee for extraordinary circumstances.

Evaluation criteria
A 4-part admission procedure is used, including evaluation of science grades, evaluation of all 3 GRE® scores, assessment of the application and narrative, and a personal interview.

Prerequisite science GPA	30%
Test scores	40%
Interview score including:	30%
References	
Animal/veterinary experience	
Leadership in college and community	
Autobiographical essay	

Admitted Fall 2012

	Number of Applicants	Number of New Entrants
Resident	119	45
Nonresident	1,156	63
North Dakota	15	4
Total:	1,290	112

* For further information, see the listing of contracting states and provinces.

Expenses for the 2012–2013 Academic Year

Tuition and fees (subject to change)
Resident	$22,403.60
Nonresident	$48,897.20

* For further information, see the listing of contracting states and provinces.

Dual-Degree Programs

Combined DVM–graduate degree programs are available.
Combined DVM-MPH degree programs are available.

Early Admission Program

The Veterinary Scholars Early Admission Program is designed for those students having a genuine desire to enter the veterinary profession who attend Kansas State University with an ACT score of 29 or greater or an equivalent SAT score and who complete a successful interview during the fall semester of their freshman undergraduate year.

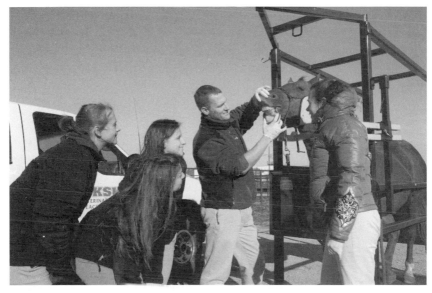

Veterinary students assist with an equine exam as part of their studies. Photo by David Adams, Kansas State University College of Veterinary Medicine.

Louisiana State University

Office of Student and Academic Affairs
School of Veterinary Medicine
Louisiana State University
Skip Bertman Drive
Baton Rouge LA 70803
Telephone: (225) 578-9537
Fax: (225) 578-9546
Email: svmadmissions@lsu.edu
www.vetmed.lsu.edu/admissions

The Louisiana State University campus is located in Baton Rouge, which has a population of more than 500,000 and is a major industrial city, a thriving port, and the state's capital. Since it is located on the Mississippi River, Baton Rouge was a target for domination by Spanish, French, and English settlers. The city bears the influence of all three cultures and offers a range of choices in everything from food to architectural design. Geographically, Baton Rouge is the center of south Louisiana's main cultural and recreational attractions. Equally distant from New Orleans and the fabled Cajun bayou country, there is an abundance of cultural and outdoor recreational activities. South Louisiana has a balmy climate that encourages lush vegetation and comfortable temperatures year round.

The campus encompasses more than 2,000 acres in the southern part of Baton Rouge and is bordered on the west by the Mississippi River. The Veterinary Medicine Building, occupied in 1978, houses the academic departments, the veterinary library, and the Veterinary Teaching Hospital and Clinics. The school is fully accredited by the American Veterinary Medical Association.

Application Information

For specific application information (availability, deadlines, fees, and VMCAS participation), please refer to the LSU SVM admissions website at www.vetmed.lsu.edu/admissions.

Residency implications: The LSU SVM accepts 55-60 in-state residents and has approximately 9 seats reserved for AR contract students. The remaining 18-23 seats are offered to non-resident students.

Prerequisites for Admission

Course requirements and semester hours
General Biology	8
Microbiology (w/lab)[1]	4
Physics	6

General Chemistry	8
Organic Chemistry	3
Biochemistry[2]	3
English Composition	6
Speech Communication	3
Mathematics	5
Electives	20

[1]Lab component must accompany the microbiology lecture.
[2]Must have organic chemistry as prerequisite. For more details regarding prerequisites, visit the LSU SVM Admissions web site at www.vetmed.lsu.edu/admissions

Required undergraduate GPA: the minimum acceptable GPA for required coursework is 3.00 on a 4.00 scale. The mean GPA of the most recent entering class at the time of acceptance was 3.77.

AP credit policy: must appear on official college transcripts and be equivalent to the appropriate college-level coursework.

Course completion deadline: prerequisite courses must be completed by the end of the spring term preceding matriculation. (For example, if applying for fall '14 matriculation, all prerequisites must be completed by the end of the spring '14 semester.)

Standardized examinations: The GRE® revised General Test is required. The scores must be received no later than November 15. NOTE - All applicants must take the GRE® revised General Test that started in August '11. The old, General GRE® exam is NOT acceptable beginning in the 2012 - 2013 application cycle.

Additional requirements and considerations
Animal/veterinary work experience is highly desired along with motivation, maturity, leadership skills; demonstrated communication skills; breadth of interests; entrepreneurial and business skills.

International students are accepted only if all prerequisite coursework is completed at an accredited university within the United States or Canada.

Summary of Admission Procedure

Timetable
    Last date to take GRE: October 1
    VMCAS application deadline: Wednesday, October 2, 2013 at 1:00 p m.
      Eastern Time

Supplemental application deadline: November 15 (Supplemental
   Application Link: www.vetmed.lsu.edu/admissions)
Supplemental application fee ($75) deadline: November 15
GRE® score submission deadline: November 15
Date interviews are held: February/March*
Date acceptances mailed: mid-March
School begins: mid-August
*Interview invitations are extended to a select number of Louisiana,
   Arkansas, and out of state applicants as determined by the LSU
   SVM Admissions Committee.

Deposit (to hold place in class): $500.00 for nonresidents only.

Deferments: considered on a case-by-case basis.

Evaluation criteria
The approximate components of the evaluation scoring are:
   Objective evaluation:
      GPA required courses   29%
      GPA last 45 hours   18%
      Test scores   18%
   Subjective evaluation:
      Animal/veterinary experience, references   15%
         (min. of 3 required, one by a veterinarian),
   essay, knowledge of profession, etc
      Personal interview   10%
      Committee evaluation   10%

2012–2013 Admissions Summary

	Number of Applicants	Number of New Entrants
Resident	154	63
Contract (AR)	39	9
Nonresident	553	13
Total:	798	88

Expenses for the 2012–2013 Academic Year

Tuition and fees (estimated)
   Resident $19,552
   Nonresident
      Contract* $19,552
      Other nonresident $45,352

* For further information, see the listing of contracting states and provinces.

Michigan State University

Office of Admissions
College of Veterinary Medicine
Veterinary Medical Center
784 Wilson Road, F-110
East Lansing MI 48824
Telephone: (517) 353-9793; fax: (517) 353-3041;
Email: admiss@cvm.msu.edu
www.cvm.msu.edu

Michigan State University's campus is bordered by the city of East Lansing, which offers sidewalk cafes, restaurants, shops, and convenient mass transit. The campus is traversed by the Red Cedar River and has many miles of bike paths and walkways. This park-like setting provides an ideal venue in which MSU's 48,906 students may enjoy outdoor concerts and plays, canoeing, and cross-country skiing. The campus is located in East Lansing, three miles east of Michigan's capitol in Lansing. It sits on a 5,200-acre campus with 2,100 acres in existing or planned development. There are 532 buildings which include 103 academic buildings.

The college is a national leader in state-of-the-art technology and facilities. The Information Technology Center empowers and assists students, faculty, and staff with the knowledge needed to fulfill everyday computer tasks. The Veterinary Teaching Hospital has one of the largest caseloads in the country. Outstanding faculty are involved in teaching veterinary students, providing patient treatment and diagnostic services, and conducting veterinary research.

There are four state-of-the art facilities that have been added in the past few years to our medical complex. They are the new Diagnostic Center for Population and Animal Health (DCPAH), the Center for Comparative Oncology, the Mary Anne McPhail Equine Performance Center, and the Matilda R. Wilson Pegasus Critical Care Center and the Training Center for Dairy Professionals. For information about these centers, please visit the links provided below.

http://animalhealth.msu.edu/
http://cvm.msu.edu/hospital/services/comparative-oncology-center
http://cvm.msu.edu/hospital/special-facilities/Plone//research/
    research-centers/mcphail-equine-performance-center
http://cvm.msu.edu/departments/large-animal-clinical-sciences/
    services-research-centers/pegasus-critical-care-center?
    searchterm=pegasus

Application Information

For specific application information (pre-requisite science courses, deadlines, fees, and VMCAS participation), please refer to our website http://cvm.msu.edu

Residency implications: priority is given to Michigan residents. Up to 35 positions are filled with nonresident and international applicants.

Prerequisites for Admission

Course requirements and semester hours
General education

English composition	3
Social and behavioral sciences	6
Humanities	6

Mathematics and biological and physical sciences

General inorganic chemistry (with laboratory)	3
Organic chemistry (with laboratory)	6
Biochemistry (upper-division)	3
General biology (with laboratory)	6
College algebra and trigonometry	3
College physics (with laboratory)	8
Nutrition	3
Genetics	3
Cell biology (eukaryotic)	3
Microbiology (with laboratory)	4

Required undergraduate GPA: No minimum required. The mean cumulative GPA for the entering class (2012) was 3.70 on a 4.00 scale.

AP credit policy: AP credit(s) must appear on an official transcript and be equivalent to appropriate college-level coursework.

Course completion deadline: For those applying summer 2013, all prerequisite courses must be completed by the end of spring semester, 2014

Standardized examinations: The Graduate Record Examination (GRE®), general test, is required to be taken no later than September 30. Test scores older than 5 years will not be accepted. For the class entering in 2012, average GRE scores were: 1201 combined verbal and quantitative. The Test of English as a Foreign Language (TOEFL) is required for applicants whose primary language is not English.

Additional Requirements and Considerations
- Evaluation of written application (including veterinary/research experience)
- Supplemental application. A link to the supplemental application will be sent to the applicant
- Letters of recommendation (3 submitted by October 2, 2013 at 1:00 p.m. Eastern Time through VMCAS; 1 must be completed by a veterinarian)
- Interview (by the discretion of the Committee on Student Admissions)

Summary of Admission Procedure

Timetable

VMCAS application deadline: Wednesday, October 2, 2013 at 1:00 p.m. Eastern Time

Electronic evaluations to VMCAS: Wednesday, October 2, 2013 at 1:00 p.m. Eastern Time

GRE taken by September 30. The dateline to received GRE scores is December 15

All transcripts submitted to MSUCVM by October 2 (postmarked date)

International transcripts must be evaluated by a translation service such as World Education Services (WES), Josef Silny or the American Association of Collegiate Registrars and Admissions Officers, Foreign Education Credential Service (AACRAO). It is recommended that transcript(s) be submitted to the translation service at least one month prior to the deadline of October 2

Deposit (to hold place in class): (nonrefundable) $500.00 for residents; $1,000.00 for nonresidents.

Deferments: are rare.

2012–2013 admissions summary

	Number of Applicants	Number of New Entrants
Resident	198	76
Nonresident/International	587	35
Total:	785	111

Expenses for the 2011–2012 Academic Year

Tuition and fees

Resident	$26,016
Nonresident	$52,206

Early Admission Program

The Veterinary Scholars Admission Program has been established by the College of Veterinary Medicine in cooperation with the Honors College at Michigan State. This program provides an admission opportunity for students who wish to enter the four year professional veterinary medicine degree program after earning a bachelor's degree. The bachelor's degree program must include advanced and enriched coursework representing scholarly interest and achievements. Enrollment at MSU and membership in the Honors College are required to be eligible for this option. For information on Honors College membership, contact: Honors College, 105 Eustace-Hall, 468 E. Circle Drive, Michigan State University, East Lansing, MI 48824; telephone (517) 355-2326; or visit their website at http://honorscollege.msu.edu/.

Production Medicine Scholars Pathway

The Production Medicine Scholars Pathway has been established by the College of Veterinary Medicine in cooperation with the department of Animal Science at Michigan State University. This pathway is available to MSU Animal Science students who complete, in addition to the minimum pre-veterinary medicine requirements, a bachelor's degree in Animal Science with a concentration in production animal medicine. The concentration is designed to prepare students for a career in herd based, agricultural veterinary practice. The pathway provides an early admission option for Michigan State University students planning to earn a baccalaureate degree in animal science with a concentration in production medicine. Successful applicants must have strong academic and non-academic credentials and a demonstrated interest in food animal production medicine and agricultural veterinary practice. Additional information about the pathway may be obtained from 1250 Anthony Hall, 474 S. Shaw Lane, Department of Animal Science, Michigan State University, East Lansing, MI 48824 or visit the website http://www.ans.msu.edu/

Dual Degree Programs

Combined DVM – MPH degree program available

Combined online DVM/ MS in Food Safety available

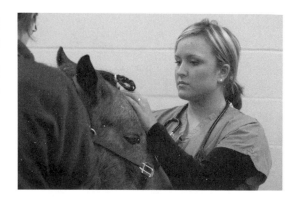

University of Minnesota

Office of Academic and Student Affairs
College of Veterinary Medicine
108 Pomeroy Center
1964 Fitch Ave.
University of Minnesota
St. Paul MN 55108
Telephone: (612) 624-4747
Email: dvminfo@umn.edu
www.cvm.umn.edu

The University of Minnesota College of Veterinary Medicine prepares future leaders in companion animal, food animal, and public health practice, as well as research and education. University of Minnesota students benefit from one of the largest teaching hospitals in the country, as well as world renowned faculty in zoonotic diseases, comparative medicine, and population systems. The College offers state-of-the-art facilities, including the Veterinary Medical Center, Leatherdale Equine Center, and the Raptor Center, which in 1988 became the world's first facility designed specifically for birds of prey. Off-site facilities include farms throughout Minnesota and around the world.

The College of Veterinary Medicine is located on the 540-acre St. Paul campus. Students enjoy a small, intimate campus atmosphere of approximately 3,000 students while benefiting from the numerous amenities available within one of the nation's largest university systems.

The Twin Cities of Minneapolis and St. Paul have a combined population of approximately 2.5 million people and represents one of the largest metropolitan areas where a veterinary college is located. The Twin Cities is the cultural center for the region, abundant with outdoor recreational opportunities, and is repeatedly cited as one of the most livable metropolitan areas in the nation.

During the first three years of the D.V.M. program, students focus on the study of the normal animal, the pathogenesis of diseases and the prevention, alleviation and clinical therapy of diseases. Students gain hands-on experience throughout the entire program in clinical and professional skills courses.

The program concludes with thirteen months of clinical rotations in the Veterinary Medical Center, during which time students learn methods of veterinary care and develop skills needed for professional practice. Students can choose from over 80 rotation offerings. The fourth year includes up to twelve weeks of externship experiences at off-campus sites of the student's choice.

Application Information

Application requirements include a complete VMCAS application, three electronic letters of reference submitted through VMCAS, official transcripts submitted through VMCAS, GRE examination scores, and an $80 application processing fee. The University of Minnesota College of Veterinary Medicine does not utilize a supplemental application.

The application, transcripts, and references are due to VMCAS by their respective deadlines.

All other application materials are due to the College by the application deadline of October 2, 2013 at 1 p.m. Eastern Time.

For more application information, please visit http://www.cvm.umn.edu/education/prospective/home.html .

Residency implications: first priority is given to residents of Minnesota and residents of states/provinces with which a reciprocity or contract agreement exists (North Dakota and South Dakota). Residents of other states are encouraged to apply. International applicants are only considered if their pre-veterinary courses have been completed at a U.S. or Canadian college or university.

The University of Minnesota will accept 100 students into the program each year. Approximately 55 of the 100 seats are reserved for resident/reciprocity eligible applicants. Approximately 45 seats are held for non-resident applicants.

Prerequisites for Admission

Course requirements and semester hours

Freshman English, communication	6–10
Mathematics	3–5
Chemistry (with laboratory)	
General inorganic	6–10
General organic*	3–5
Biology (with laboratory)	3–5
Zoology/animal biology (with laboratory)	3–5
Physics (with laboratory)	6–10
Biochemistry	3–5
Genetics	3–5
Microbiology (with laboratory)	3–5
Liberal education	12–16

* Two quarters with one laboratory or one semester with laboratory

All prerequisites must be graded at a C- or better. Math and science prerequisites courses must be recent within 10 years.

A minimum of 4 courses from the following areas of study: anthropology, art, economics, geography, history, humanities, literature (including foreign language literature), music, political science, psychology, public speaking, social science, sociology, theater.

Required undergraduate GPA: 2.75 minimum GPA required. The class of 2016 had a mean GPA of 3.63 (on a 4.00 scale) for required courses and 3.72 for the last 60 quarter-hour or 45 semester-hour credits of coursework prior to admission.

AP credit policy: must appear on official college transcripts and be equivalent to the appropriate college-level coursework.

Course completion deadline: prerequisite courses must be completed by the end of the spring term (not later than June 15) of the academic year in which application is made. No more than five prerequisite science courses may be pending completion during the fall and spring semesters of the application cycle. Science laboratory courses are not included in the count of five.

Standardized examinations: Graduate Record Examination (GRE®), general test, is required. Results must be received by the College by the application deadline. The mean combined score for the verbal and quantitative sections of the GRE for the class of 2016 was 1200. When scheduling your exam, confirm your test date will allow enough time for results to be delivered by the application deadline. Send test results to institution code 6904.

Summary of Admission Procedure

Timetable
> VMCAS application deadline: Wednesday, October 2, 2013 at 1:00 p.m. Eastern Time
> Date acceptances mailed: Late February
> School begins: early September

Deposit (to hold place in class): $500.00.

Deferments: can be requested for extenuating circumstances that warrant a 1-year delay in admission. Requests to defer submitted after July 15 will not be considered.

Evaluation criteria
> *Objective measures of educational background*
>> GPA in required courses
>> GPA in recent courses
>> Test scores
> *Behavioral interviews*

Subjective measures of personal experience
Employment record
Extracurricular and/or community service activities
Leadership abilities
References
Maturity/reliability
Animal/veterinary knowledge, experience, and interest

2011–2012 admissions summary

	Number of Applicants	Number of New Entrants
Resident*	189	55
Nonresident	759	45
Total:	948	100

The figures for new entrants include students taking delayed admission from the previous year.

*Includes residents of North and South Dakota and Manitoba.

Expenses for the 2011–2012 Academic Year

Tuition and fees

Residents	$32,456*
Nonresidents	$56,210*

* This includes all tuition and fees

Students from Minnesota and South Dakota pay resident tuition rates. Students from North Dakota can apply to the state of North Dakota for a contract seat. Approved North Dakota students pay resident tuition rates. North Dakota students not approved pay non-resident tuition rates. Students from all other states or international locations pay non-resident tuition rates.

The University of Minnesota Raptor Center rehabilitates more than 700 sick and injured raptors each year, while helping to identify emerging environmental issues related to raptor health and populations. The Raptor Center reaches more than 200,000 people annually through its unique public education programs and events and trains veterinary students and veterinarians from around the world.

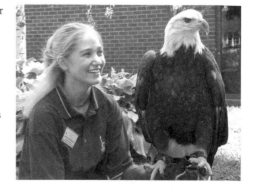

Mississippi State University

Office of Student Admissions
College of Veterinary Medicine
P.O. Box 6100
Mississippi State University
Mississippi State MS 39762
Telephone: (662) 325-9065 or 325-4161
Email: MSU-CVMAdmissions@cvm.msstate.edu
www.cvm.msstate.edu

Starkville is home to more than 20,000 MSU students and their Bulldogs. Starkville is located in northeast central Mississippi and has a population of 24,000. Being a land-grant university, MSU is green and beautifully landscaped. The university includes 9 farms scattered throughout the state. The College of Veterinary Medicine (the Wise Center) was completed in 1982. The college includes 620 rooms on 8 acres, or 360,000 square feet, under one roof.

The curriculum of the MSU-CVM is divided into 2 phases: Phase 1 (freshman and sophomore years) and Phase 2 (junior and senior years).

- Year 1 uses foundation courses to expose the student to important medical concepts and address multidisciplinary problems.

- Year 2 is devoted to the study of clinical diseases and abnormalities of animal species. Surgery labs begin in the second year.

- Year 3 is comprised of clinical rotations in the College's Animal Health Center, and elective courses.

- Year 4 includes core rotations in internal medicine and ICU, large animal ambulatory and the Jackson Emergency/Referral Clinic. The remainder of the year is largely experiential and offers the student the opportunity to select among approved experiences in advanced clinical rotations, elective courses, or externships.

The first 3 years of the curriculum are 9–10 months in length, while the fourth year is 12 months.

Application Information

For specific application information (availability, deadlines, fees, and VMCAS participation), please refer to the contact information listed above.

Residency implications: Mississippi State accepts 40 Mississippi residents, 5 contract students from both South Carolina and West Virginia, and 35 non-resident applicants.

Prerequisites for Admission

Course requirements and semester hours

English composition	6
Speech or Technical Writing	3
Mathematics (college algebra or higher) *	6
General biology with laboratory	8
Microbiology with laboratory*	4
General chemistry with laboratories*	8
Organic chemistry with laboratories*	8
Biochemistry*	3
Physics (may be trig-based) *	6
Advanced (upper level) science electives*	12
Humanities, fine arts, social and behavioral sciences	15

* Science and mathematics courses must be completed or updated within six calendar years prior to the anticipated date of enrollment.

Required undergraduate GPA: At the time of application, a minimum GPA of 2.8 on a 4.0 scale overall and in required math/science courses. No grade lower than a C- is acceptable in any required course. Minimum GPA must be maintained throughout the application process. The class of 2016 has an average undergraduate GPA of 3.60.

AP credit policy: must appear on official college transcripts and be equivalent to the appropriate college-level coursework.

Course completion deadline: prerequisites must be completed by the end of the spring term prior to fall matriculation into the first-year class.

Standardized examinations: Graduate Record Exam (GRE®), general test, is required (no minimum score) and is due at the school by October 1.

New test: Students should schedule the GRE exam 30 days prior to the deadline.

Additional requirements and considerations

> Evaluation of written application
> Supplemental application and fee (http://www.cvm.msstate.edu/ academics/student_admissions.html)
> Letters of recommendation (3 submitted through VMCAS; 1 must be completed by a veterinarian)
> Interview (by invitation on a competitive basis)

Summary of Admission Procedure

Timetable
> VMCAS application deadline: Wednesday, October 2, 2013 at 1:00 p.m.
> Eastern Time
> Date interviews are held: February
> Date acceptances mailed: February or March
> First-year classes begin: early July

Deposit (to hold place in class): $500.00.

Deferments: requests are considered on an individual basis.

Evaluation criteria
> Grades
> Quality of academic program
> Test scores
> Animal/veterinary experience
> Interview
> References (3 required, one by a veterinarian)
> Application (includes personal statement)

Class of 2016 admissions summary

	Number of Applicants	Number of New Entrants
Resident	92*	40*
Nonresident	881*	45*
Total:	973*	85*

*Includes students admitted through the Early Entry Program

Expenses for the 2012–2013 Academic Year

Tuition and fees

Resident and contract seats	$18,011
Nonresident	$43,011

Dual-Degree Programs

Combined DVM–graduate degree programs are available.

International Students

International students are accepted

University of Missouri

Office of Academic Affairs
College of Veterinary Medicine
W203 Veterinary Medicine Building
University of Missouri-Columbia
Columbia MO 65211
Telephone: (573) 884-3341
Email: seayk@missouri.edu
https://cvmsecure.missouri.edu/admission_application/

The University of Missouri is located among rolling forested hills north of the famous Lake of the Ozarks. Columbia is noted for its high quality of life and low cost of living and is consistently rated among the best cities to live in by Money Magazine. The city abounds with walking trails, 3,000 acres of state park lands, federal forests, and wildlife refuges. Columbia is located between Kansas City and St. Louis—cities that have major-league sports teams and other big-city recreational amenities. Columbia itself offers SEC football, basketball, baseball and other sports. It boasts a 65,000-seat stadium, several 18-hole golf courses, and other indoor and outdoor recreation facilities. Our location near a metropolitan area provides a strong primary and referral small animal case load. Columbia's proximity to rural central Missouri results in an exceptional food animal and equine case load.

MU, a major research university with 34,000 students, consists of 19 schools and colleges located on a 1,335-acre campus. The College of Veterinary Medicine is noted for its unique curriculum that gives students 2 years of undiluted clinical experience before graduation as opposed to the traditional 1–1½ years. Students benefit from exposure to specialty medical areas such as clinical cardiology, neurology, orthopedics, ophthalmology, and oncology. Students also gain experience with advanced equipment such as a linear accelerator for treatment of cancer, PET Scanner, MRI, state-of-the-art ultrasonography, extensive endoscopy equipment, cold lasers, a surgery room C-arm for radiography during surgical procedures, and others. MU is unique in having a medical school, nursing school, school of health related professions, state cancer research center, the life sciences center and department of animal science on the same campus, thus enhancing teaching, research, and clinical services.

Application Information

All applicants must use VMCAS and submit our Supplemental Application. For specific application information (availability, deadlines, fees, and VMCAS participation), please refer to the contact information listed above.

Supplemental Application: Available at www.cvm.missouri.edu between July 1 and Oct 1.

Residency implications: sixty seats are given to Missouri and sixty to non-residents. A total of 120 seats awarded each year.

Prerequisites for Admission

Course requirements and semester hours

English or communication	6
College algebra or more advanced mathematics	3
Physics	5
Biological science	10
Social sciences or humanities	10
Biochemistry (Organic Chemistry pre-req.)	3
Minimum credit hours	**60**

Required undergraduate GPA: Applicants must have a cumulative GPA of 3.00 or more on a 4.00 scale. The most recent entering class had a mean GPA of 3.77 at the time of acceptance.

AP credit policy: must appear on official college transcript and be equivalent to the appropriate college-level coursework.

Course completion deadline: prerequisite courses must be completed by the end of the winter semester or spring quarter of the year of entry. Only two courses being used to fulfill course pre-requisites may be pending completion in the spring/winter semester prior to matriculation.

Standardized examinations: The Medical College Admission Test (MCAT) or the Graduate Record Examination (GRE®) general test is required. Test scores older than 3 years will not be accepted. Exams must be taken prior to January 1, 2014 and scores submitted by February 1, 2014.

Additional requirements and considerations

Animal/veterinary experience
Recommendations/evaluations (3 required)
  Employer
  Academic advisors/faculty member
  Veterinarians
Extracurricular and/or community service activities
Essays
  Animal experience
  Explanation of choice of veterinary medicine as a profession
Employment history

Summary of Admission Procedure

Timetable
> VMCAS application deadline: Wednesday, October 2, 2013 at 1:00 p.m. Eastern Time
> Date interviews are held: February–March (late December–early January for non-residents)
> Date acceptances mailed: mid-April
> School begins: late August

Deposit (to hold place in class): $100.00 for residents; $500.00 for nonresidents.

Deferments: each is considered individually by the admissions committee.

Evaluation criteria
The admission process consists of a preliminary file review of all applicants. Personal interviews are subsequently granted to all qualified Missouri residents and 225 to 250 nonresidents.

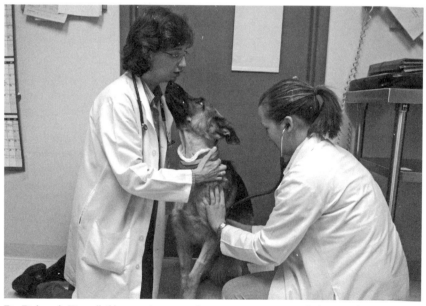

Dr. Deborah Fine, (left) an assistant professor in veterinary cardiology at the University of Missouri College of Veterinary Medicine, supervises a student examining a patient at the Veterinary Medical Teaching Hospital. Spending nearly two years in a clinical instruction setting gives MU CVM students the opportunity to acquire hands-on experience in several specialty areas of small animal medicine, including cardiology, orthopaedics, ophthalmology, oncology, radiology and community medicine, as well as food animal and equine medicine, as part of their professional curriculum.

	% weight
Grades	35
Test scores	5
Interview score including:	60

Animal/veterinary experience
Interpersonal skills
Work ethic
Leadership in college and community
Life experiences and diversity

2011–2012 admissions summary

	Number of Applicants	Number of New Entrants
Resident	140	60
Nonresident	809	60
Total:	949	120

Expenses for the 2012–2013 Academic Year (Updates for 2013-2014 available June 2013)

Students who attend the University of Missouri have the option of applying for Missouri residency after year 1. If residency is approved, the student will pay non-resident tuition in year 1 only.

Tuition and fees

Resident	$20,092
Nonresident	$49,398

Students who attend the University of Missouri have the option of applying for Missouri residency after Year 1. If approved, then the students will pay nonresident tuition in Year 1 only.

Dual-Degree Programs

Combined DVM–graduate degree programs are available.

Early Admission Program

The Pre-veterinary Medicine and AgScholars Programs guarantee acceptance into the professional program upon satisfactory completion of the undergraduate requirements. Eligibility requires a high-school senior or University of Missouri freshman to have a composite ACT score of at least 30 and 27 respectively, or an equivalent SAT score. Eligible applicants will be interviewed, and a satisfactory score must be achieved to become a Scholar. Selected veterinary medical faculty will be assigned as mentors. Scholars receive priority consideration for part-time employment in the college. Further information may be obtained by contacting the Office of Academic Affairs.

North Carolina State University

Student Services Office
College of Veterinary Medicine
North Carolina State University
1060 William Moore Drive, Box 8401
Raleigh NC 27607
Telephone: (919) 513-6262
Email: cvm_dvm@ncsu.edu
www.cvm.ncsu.edu

The North Carolina State University College of Veterinary Medicine is located on a 182-acre site in Raleigh, the state capital, which has a population of more than 400,000. The sandy shores of North Carolina's beautiful coastline are a short ride to the east, and the Great Smoky Mountains are to the west. The climate includes mild winters and warm summers.

The College of Veterinary Medicine opened in the fall of 1981 and encompasses 20 buildings on the main Centennial Biomedical Campus, including a teaching hospital, classrooms, animal wards, research and teaching laboratories, and an audiovisual area. The college has 140 faculty members and a capacity for 400 veterinary medical students with training for interns, residents, and graduate students.

Construction started fall 2002 on the Centennial Biomedical Campus, which will be anchored by the College of Veterinary Medicine. An extension of the original NCSU Centennial Campus concept, the Centennial Biomedical Campus will house approximately 32 building sites. It will include an additional 1.6 million square feet of space over the next 20 years, resulting in a five-fold expansion of the current college and teaching hospital. The two-year construction of the Randall B. Terry, Jr. Companion Animal Veterinary Medical Center was completed in June 2011. The Terry Center is considered the national model for excellence in companion animal medicine. The Terry Center offers cutting-edge technologies for imaging, cardiac care, cancer treatments, internal medicine, and surgery; has more than double the size of the former companion animal hospital; and accommodates the more than 20,000 cases referred to the CVM each year.

The Centennial Biomedical Campus will emphasize partnerships that work to bring academia, government and industry together. The focus of this campus is on biomedical applications, both to animals and humans. It will provide opportunities for industry and government researchers, entrepreneurs, clinical trial companies, as well as collaborations with other universities to work side by side with faculty and students at the College of Veterinary Medicine.

Application Information

For specific application information (availability, deadlines, fees, and VMCAS participation), please refer to the contact information listed above.

Residency implications: priority is given to North Carolina residents.

NOTE: The college increased its incoming class size from 80 to 100 starting with the 2012 admissions cycle. The exact slot allocation between residents and nonresidents has yet to be determined. The previous allocation was 62 resident and 18 nonresident slots.

NC State does accept international applicants.

Prerequisites for Admission

Course requirements and semester hours

Any combination of English Composition I, English Composition II, Public Speaking, or Communication	6
College Calculus	3
Introduction to Statistics	3
General Physics I, II (with laboratory)	8
General Chemistry I, II (with laboratory)	8
Organic Chemistry I, II (with laboratory)	8
General Biology (with laboratory)	4
Principles of Genetics	4
General Microbiology (with laboratory)	4
Biochemistry	3
Social Sciences and Humanities	6
Animal Nutrition	3

AP credit policy: must appear on official college transcripts with course name and credit hours and be equivalent to the appropriate college-level coursework.

Course completion deadline: only 2 courses may be pending completion in the spring semester, and both must be completed (with transcript evidence) by the end of the spring semester prior to matriculation. Pending courses (including correspondence courses) may not be completed in the summer session immediately preceding matriculation.

Standardized examinations: Graduate Record Examination (GRE®), general test, is required. The scores must be received by the October 2 application deadline.

There is no deadline to take the GRE; only a deadline to submit scores. However, we do recommend that applicants take the GRE by September 1 in order for the scores to arrive by the deadline.

Additional requirements and considerations
>Animal/veterinary knowledge, experience, motivation, and maturity
>Personal statement
>Recommendations/evaluations (3 required; at least 2 from
>>veterinarians/scientists with whom applicant has worked is highly
>>recommended)
>Extracurricular activities

Summary of Admission Procedure

Timetable
>VMCAS application deadline: Wednesday, October 2, 2013 at 1:00 p.m.
>>Eastern Time (VMCAS and NC State supplemental)
>Date acceptances mailed: no later than April 1
>School begins: August

Deposit (to hold place in class): $250.00.

Deferments: are considered for 1 year only, subject to Admissions Committee approval.

Evaluation criteria
Selection for admission is a 2-phase process:

Phase 1—Objective criteria:
>Required course GPA: 3.3 Resident, 3.4 Nonresident
>Cumulative GPA: 3.0 Resident, 3.4 Nonresident
>GPA in last 45+ credits attempted: 3.3 Resident, 3.4 Nonresident
>GRE test score
>Supplemental Application

Phase 2—Subjective score:
>Applicant folder review by admissions committee

2011–2012 admissions summary

	Number of Applicants	Number of New Entrants*
Resident	189	80
Nonresident	648	20
Total:	837	100

* Estimated

Expenses for the 2012–2013 Academic Year

Tuition and fees
Resident	$15,377.56
Nonresident	$38,140.56

Dual Degree Programs

Combined DVM–graduate degree programs are available.

Early Admission Program

Two special admissions options are available: (1) for North Carolina residents focusing on swine, poultry, or food animal medicine in concert with the College of Agriculture and Life Sciences, and (2) for students focusing on laboratory animal medicine in concert with the College of Agriculture at North Carolina A&T State University.

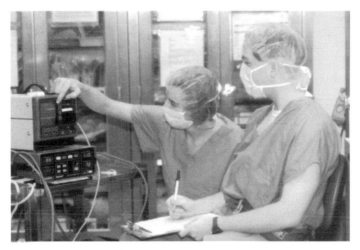

Veterinary students monitor the vital signs of a patient during surgery at the North Carolina State University Veterinary Teaching Hospital. Photo courtesy of North Carolina State University College of Veterinary Medicine.

The Ohio State University

Office of Student Affairs
College of Veterinary Medicine
Suite 127 Veterinary Medicine Academic Building
1900 Coffey Road
The Ohio State University
Columbus OH 43210-1089
Telephone: (614) 247-1512
Fax: (614) 292-6989
Email: prospective@cvm.osu.edu
www.vet.ohio-state.edu

The Ohio State University is located in Columbus, the state's capital and the nation's 15th largest city. Columbus has been rated the 7th best city in the nation for cost of living (Forbes Magazine) and one of the country's top-10 places to live (Money). Columbus offers all the cultural perks you would expect from a major metropolitan area including the #1 zoo in the country, according to the USA Travel Guide.

The Ohio State University was founded in 1870 and is one of the nation's leading academic centers, consistently ranks as Ohio's best, and one of the nation's top-20 public universities. The campus consists of thousands of acres, hundreds of buildings, more than 15,000 faculty and staff, and more than 56,000 students.

The Veterinary Medical Center includes a Hospital for Companion Animals, Food Animal, and the Galbreath Equine Center. The patient load is one of the highest in the country and farmlands can be accessed 10 miles from campus. The Veterinary Medicine Academic Building has nearly 10,000 square feet of space and includes research labs, classrooms, a library, computer lab, and academic offices.

The Ohio State College of Veterinary Medicine is part of one of the largest and most comprehensive health sciences centers in the country that includes dentistry, medicine, nursing, optometry, pharmacy, public health, and veterinary medicine.

Application Information

For specific application information (availability, deadlines, fees, and VMCAS participation), please refer to the contact information listed above.

Residency implications: 162 new students are accepted each year. Applicants from all states will be considered. In-state and out-of-state applicants are given equal consideration. International applicants are considered.

Prerequisites for Admission

For the humanities and social sciences requirement, students are encouraged to elect the courses required for the bachelor of science curriculum. Courses in communication, journalism, sociology, economics, and animal behavior are strongly recommended. Elective courses are at the student's discretion after consultation with an advisor. However, highly recommended electives include embryology, histology, cell biology, immunology, anatomy, physiology, and animal science including nutrition

Students enrolled in the preveterinary medicine curriculum are encouraged to take electives that will provide a well-rounded education in addition to those biological sciences preparatory to the veterinary medical curriculum.

Course requirements	Semester units	Quarter units
English	3	5
General chemistry (with laboratory)*	10	15
Organic chemistry*	8	6
Biochemistry*	5	5
Biology*	8	10
Genetics*	3	5
Microbiology (with laboratory)*	4	5
Mathematics (algebra and trigonometry)	5	5
General physics (with laboratory)*	10	10
Humanities and social sciences	14	20
Electives	8	10

* Must have been completed within the 10 years preceding the application deadline.

Required undergraduate GPA: the minimum GPA to be considered is 3.0 on a 4.0 scale. The most recent entering class had a mean overall GPA of 3.65 and a science GPA of 3.48. Prerequisite science GPA is evaluated as well as last 45 semester or quarter hours.

AP credit policy: AP credit given if course is listed on official transcript.

Course completion deadline: all but one prerequisite course must be completed by the end of the fall semester or quarter coinciding with submission of the application. The final remaining prerequisite course must be completed at the end of the following term (spring semester or winter quarter). Failure to satisfactorily complete all prerequisites with a grade of C or better will result in automatic loss of a candidate's seat in the class.

Standardized examinations: Graduate Record Examination (GRE) general test or the Medical College Admission (MCAT) test is required. Most applicants choose to take the GRE. Tests must be taken by September 30 but within five years of application. Test scores must be received no later than October 1 of the year of application. Use GRE code: 1592 and Department Code: 0617

Additional requirements and considerations
> Academic background/difficulty
> College Extracurricular Activities
> Employment/Leadership Activities/Honors & Awards
> Veterinary and Animal Experience
> References (1 must be from a veterinarian. Evaluators may not be relatives)
> Personal statement
> Interpersonal/Communication skills
> Adversity coping skills
> Knowledge and understanding of the profession

Summary of Admission Procedure

Timetable
> VMCAS application deadline: Wednesday, October 2, 2013 at 1:00 p.m. Eastern Time
> Date interviews are held: December–February
> Rolling offer: December–April
> School begins: late August

Deposit (to hold place in class): $25.00 for residents; $300.00 (non-refundable fee) for contract and nonresident applicants.

Deferments: not considered.

Evaluation criteria

	% weight
File Review	30%
Objective Score	35%
Subjective Score	35%

* Applicants are interviewed and evaluated by the Admissions Committee. The interview covers subjective areas such as communication/interpersonal skills, veterinary and animal experience, knowledge and understanding of the profession. Those applicants with the highest overall evaluation are selected for the entering class.

2012–2013 admissions summary

	Number of Applicants	Number of New Entrants
Resident	217	98
Nonresident	601	66
Total:	818	164

Expenses for the 2012–2013 Academic Year

Estimated tuition and fees (subject to change)

Resident	$28,620
Nonresident*	$62,084

* For tuition purposes, **nonresident students can apply for residency after completing their first year at Ohio State.**

Summer Research Program

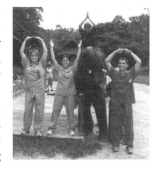

Dr. Nongnuch Inpanbutr, professor in the Department of Veterinary Biosciences is a tireless advocate for expanding students' cultural horizons. For the past several summers, Dr. Inpanbutr has taken veterinary students to Thailand to study elephant health and behavior.

The program enables students to develop scientific knowledge and skills in veterinary and comparative medicine and related research problems. Participants earn a stipend while conducting original research.

First-and second-year DVM students who are accepted into the Summer Scholar Research Program experience a laboratory setting, attend seminars, participate in field trips, travel to a national meeting, and develop new relationships with fellow students and faculty mentors.

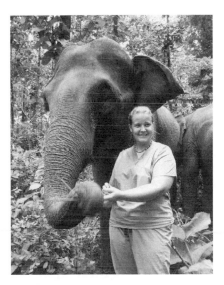

"We spent 25 days in Thailand," said then third-year OSU veterinary student Allison Lamb. "We started out in Bangkok, and then met everybody for the program at the veterinary hospital at Chian Mai University. We attended classes at the veterinary hospital to learn about elephant nutrition and behavior. The last part of the trip we spent actually going out to the different elephant camps."

Oklahoma State University

Office of Admissions
112 McElroy Hall
Center for Veterinary Health Sciences
College of Veterinary Medicine
Oklahoma State University
Stillwater OK 74078-2003
Telephone: (405) 744-6961
Fax: (405) 744-0356
Email: dvm@postoffice.cvhs.okstate.edu
www.cvhs.okstate.edu

Oklahoma State University is located in Stillwater, which has a population of about 46,000. Stillwater is in north central Oklahoma about 65 miles from Oklahoma City and 69 miles from Tulsa. The campus is exceptionally beautiful, with modified Georgian-style architecture in the new buildings. It encompasses 840 acres and more than 60 major academic buildings.

Three major buildings form the veterinary medicine complex. The oldest, McElroy Hall, houses the William E. Brock Memorial Library and Learning Center, as well as classrooms and laboratories. The Boren Veterinary Medical Teaching Hospital provides modern facilities for both academic and clinical instruction. Completing the triad is the Oklahoma Animal Disease Diagnostic Laboratory, which provides teaching resources for students in the professional curriculum and diagnostic services to Oklahoma agriculture and industry. The College of Veterinary Medicine is fully accredited by the American Veterinary Medical Association. Faculty members in the 3 academic departments share responsibility for the curriculum. These departments are Veterinary Clinical Sciences, Veterinary Pathobiology, and Physiological Sciences.

Application Information

For specific application information (availability, deadlines, fees, and VMCAS participation), please refer to the contact information listed above.

Residency implications: entering class size is 82, which includes 58 Oklahoma residents and 24 non-residents. Some non-resident contract seats are available through AR and DE. International applications are accepted.

Prerequisites for Admission

Course requirements and minimum semester hours

English composition	6
English elective	3
General chemistry (with laboratory)	8
Organic chemistry (with laboratory)	8
Biochemistry	3
Physics (Physics I & II)	8
Mathematics	3
Zoology (with laboratory)	4
Animal nutrition	3
Biological science	4
Microbiology (with laboratory)	4
Genetics	3
Humanities or social sciences	6

Required undergraduate GPA: a minimum GPA of 2.8 on a 4.00 scale is required in prerequisite courses. The mean cumulative GPA of the 2012 entering class was 3.579.

AP credit policy: AP credit accepted if documented on college transcript.

Course completion deadline: prerequisite courses must be completed by the end of the spring semester just prior to matriculation.

Standardized examinations: Graduate Record Examination (GRE®), general test is required. The class of 2016 had mean scores of 153 verbal, 150 quantitative, and analytical of 4.0. Scores must be received by December 1.

Additional requirements and considerations

Knowledge of the veterinary profession and its array of careers
Animal/veterinary work experience
Demonstrated leadership in student and/or community organizations
Three letters of recommendation, one of which must come from a
veterinarian. Other letters of reference may come from an academic
adviser, professor or other employer.

All math and science courses must have been taken within 8 years of application (courses valid up through fall 2005 for 2013-2014 application cycle).

Summary of Admission Procedure

Timetable
>VMCAS application deadline: Wednesday, October 2, 2013 at 1:00 p.m.
>>Eastern Time
>Date interviews held: February
>Date acceptances mailed: March
>School begins: mid-August

Deposit (to hold place in class): resident, $100.00; nonresident, $500.00.

Evaluation criteria
The admission procedure consists of evaluation of both academic and nonacademic criteria. The Admissions Committee considers all factors in the applicant's file, but the following are especially important: academic achievement; familiarity with the profession and sincerity of interest; recommendations; test scores; extracurricular activities; character, personality, and general fitness and commitment for a career in veterinary medicine. The committee selects those applicants considered most capable of excelling as veterinary medical students and who possess the greatest potential for success in the veterinary medical profession.

2012–2013 admissions summary

	Number of Applicants	Number of New Entrants
Resident	106	58
Nonresident	549	24
Total:	655	82

Expenses for the 2012–2013 Academic Year

Tuition and fees

Resident	$16,640
Nonresident	$36,900

Dual-Degree Programs
Combined DVM–graduate and MBA/DVM degree programs are available.

Early Admissions
The Early Admissions Program offers an admissions avenue for students entering into their first year of college and who have demonstrated exceptional academic performance, maturity and commitment to veterinary medicine and Oklahoma State University. Applicants must have an ACT score of 28 or higher and have committed to a 4-year university in Oklahoma. Further in-

formation may be obtained by contacting the Student Services Office at the address noted in previous sections.

A supplemental application is required and due on Wednesday, October 2, 2013 at 1:00 p.m. Eastern time. Application located at http://www.cvhs.okstate.edu/

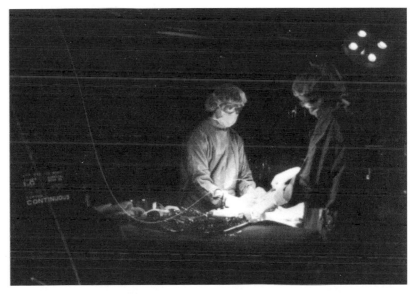

Veterinarians at Oklahoma State University's College of Veterinary Medicine perform laser surgery as part of their investigation of the medical application of lasers. Photo courtesy of the College of Veterinary Medicine, Oklahoma State University.

Oregon State University

Office of the Dean
Attention: Admissions
College of Veterinary Medicine
Oregon State University
200 Magruder Hall
Corvallis, OR 97331-4801
Telephone: (541) 737-6985
Fax: (541) 737-4245
Email: cvmadmissions@oregonstate.edu
www.oregonstate.edu/vetmed

Oregon State University (OSU) is one of only two universities in the United States to hold the Land Grant, Sea Grant, Sun Grant, and Space Grant designations, and is one of only four doctoral-granting universities in the Pacific Northwest to hold the designation of "very high research" by the Carnegie Foundation. OSU is located in Corvallis, a community of 55,000 people situated in the Willamette Valley between Portland and Eugene. Ocean beaches, lakes, rivers, forests, high desert, and the rugged Cascade and Coast Ranges are all within a 100-mile drive of Corvallis. Life in Corvallis includes lectures, concerts, films, and exhibits through the university. In the heart of the agriculturally-rich Willamette River Valley, Corvallis enjoys colorful and crisp autumns, mild and rainy winters, flowering springs, and warm, dry summers.

The first class of veterinary students entered Oregon State University in the fall of 1979, coinciding with the opening of the university's large animal hospital. Starting with the class entering in 2003, the College has offered a fully accredited, four-year program in Corvallis. The OSU College of Veterinary Medicine (CVM) supports small animal, equine, camelid, and food animal medicine and surgery as well as diagnostic and pathology services. The College opened a state-of-the-art small animal clinic in 2005 and renovation and expansion of the large animal facilities were completed in 2008. The small class size of 56 students helps to provide them with an excellent veterinary education and the opportunity to have close interaction with faculty.

Application Information

For specific application information (availability, deadlines, fees, and VMCAS participation), please refer to the contact information listed above.

Residency implications: Oregon residents and WICHE-sponsored students are eligible for resident fees. Sixteen students are accepted as nonresidents including applicants from WICHE states.

Prerequisites for Admission

Science course requirements

General biology	A course sequence of biology (2 semesters or 3 quarters).
Biological sciences	A minimum of at least 4 additional semester or 6 additional quarter credits of upper-division biological science courses with at least one laboratory.
Physics	A course sequence in physics for science majors (8 semester credits or at least 10 quarter credits).
General chemistry	A course sequence of inorganic chemistry with laboratories (2 semesters or 3 quarters).
Organic chemistry	A course sequence of organic chemistry sufficient to meet requirements for upper-division biochemistry (1-2 semesters or 2-3 quarters).
Biochemistry	A minimum of 1 semester or 2 quarters of upper-division biochemistry; a complete course sequence is preferred.
Genetics	A course in general genetics that includes both Mendelian and molecular genetics (at least 3 semester or 4 quarter credits).
Mathematics	A course or course sequence in college level algebra and trigonometry or higher level mathematics.
Physiology	A course in animal or human physiology (at least 2 semester or 3 quarter credits).
Statistics	A course(s) in statistics (at least 3 semester or 4 quarter credits).

General education course requirements

English	At least 4 semester or 6 quarter credits of English writing (e.g., English composition, technical writing).
Public speaking	At least 2 semester or 3 quarter credits of public speaking.
Humanities/social sciences	At least 8 semester or 12 quarter credits of humanities or social science courses.

These requirements will be considered met if the applicant has a bachelor's degree by July 1 of the year in which they are accepted into the program.

All prerequisite courses taken after August 2004 must be graded on an A–F scale and not taken as pass/fail. Any grade below C– in a prerequisite course is considered unsatisfactory and the course cannot be accepted to fulfill a requirement. Applicants can fulfill the requirement by repeating the same course or by substituting a higher-level course in the same field as that of the required course. A student who attends an institution that does not provide traditional grades will be evaluated on a case-by-case basis. In addition to the prerequisite courses, applicants are encouraged to take elective courses to better prepare them for the veterinary curriculum and profession. Suggested elective courses include animal science courses, business-related courses, embryology and microbiology.

Required undergraduate GPA: A minimum GPA is not required. The average cumulative GPA of admitted students is approximately 3.60.

AP credit policy: Advanced Placement (AP) and College Level Examination Program (CLEP) exam credits for lower-division prerequisite courses are accepted; credit must be reflected on the official ETS College Board score report or on an official college transcript.

Course completion deadline: Students must complete prerequisite courses by July 1 of the year in which they are accepted into the program. Complete and final official academic transcripts for all accepted applicants must be received by OSU CVM by August 1 of the year in which they are accepted into the program. It is the applicant's responsibility to verify receipt of these materials.

Standardized examinations: Graduate Record Examination (GRE®), general test, is required. The GRE must be taken within a five-year period prior to applying to veterinary school. Test scores must be received by the application deadline, October 2, 2012. It is the applicant's responsibility to verify receipt of these materials.

The Supplemental Application for the 2013-2014 Admissions Cycle, will be available the beginning of June. You will find the link to the Supplemental Application on our website at; http://oregonstate.edu/vetmed/students/future/dvm/apply. On the list of links, click on the link titled "OSU CVM Supplemental Application" if you should have any questions feel free to contact Michelle Waldron, Admissions Coordinator, at 541-737-6985 or by email at CVMAdmissions@oregonstate.edu

Additional requirements and considerations
>   Quality and rigor of academic preparation
>   Evidence of desirable skills, knowledge, attitude, and aptitude
>   Animal/veterinary knowledge and experience
>   Recommendations/evaluations (three required, at least one by a
>   veterinarian)
>   Interview (Oregon residents only)

Summary of Admission Procedure

Timetable
>   VMCAS application deadline: Wednesday, October 2, 2013 at 1:00 p.m.
>   Eastern Time
>   Supplemental application receipt deadline: October 2, 2013 at 5:00 p.m.
>   Pacific Time
>   Date interviews are held: January–February
>   Date acceptances mailed: February–March
>   School begins: late September

Deposit (to hold place in class): $50.00 for residents, $200.00 for non-residents.
Deferments: considered on an individual basis.

Evaluation criteria
Major criteria upon which applicants are selected include likelihood of academic success in the program, demonstration of qualities deemed valuable in a veterinarian, exposure to and an understanding of the veterinary profession, and contribution to diversity of the student body and the profession. Academic criteria include undergraduate and graduate grades, quantity and quality of upper-division science courses, performance in prerequisite courses, academic credit load, GRE scores, and work and/or family demands during school. Students who have taken heavy course loads (i.e. 15 or more credits per term) and performed well are likely to be better prepared for the veterinary curriculum which averages 17-21 credits per term. Nonacademic factors considered are interpersonal skills, communication skills, compassion, integrity, maturity, motivation, civic and community-mindedness, diversity of interests and activities, leadership in student and/or community organizations, scientific inquisitiveness and analytical skills. Academic and nonacademic factors are determined by evaluation of the VMCAS application, supplemental application, letters of evaluation and interview (Oregon residents only).

Oregon State University does not discriminate on the basis of race, color, gender, national origin, religion, sexual orientation, age, marital status, disability, or veteran status.

2011–2012 admissions summary

	Number of Applicants	Number of New Entrants
Resident	97	40
Contract (WICHE)*	119	1
Nonresident	338	15
Total:	554	56

* For further information, see the listing of contracting states and provinces.

Expenses for the 2012–2013 Academic Year

Tuition and fees

Resident (approximate)	$21,386
Nonresident	
Contract (WICHE)*	$21,386
Other nonresident (approximate)	$40,690

* For further information, see the listing of contracting states and provinces.

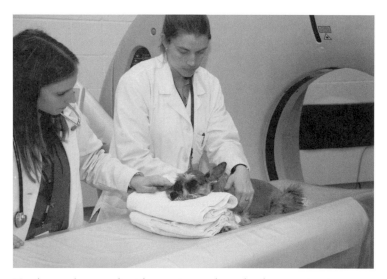

Up close and personal: with practice, students develop examination skills to deal with all sorts of patients. Photo courtesy of Oregon State University College of Veterinary Medicine.

University of Pennsylvania

Admissions Office
School of Veterinary Medicine
3800 Spruce Street University of Pennsylvania
Philadelphia PA 19104-6044
Telephone: (215) 898-5434
Fax: (215) 573-8819
Email: admissions@vet.upenn.edu
www.vet.upenn.edu

The University of Pennsylvania is located in West Philadelphia. Philadelphia is a city with a strong cultural heritage. Independence National Park includes 1 square mile of historic Philadelphia next to the Delaware River. Included are Independence Hall, the Liberty Bell, and many fine examples of colonial architecture. Philadelphia also offers theaters, museums, sports, and outdoor recreation. The Philadelphia Zoo, first in the nation, houses more than 1,600 mammals, birds, reptiles, and amphibians. The School of Veterinary Medicine enjoys a close relationship with the zoo.

The School of Veterinary Medicine was founded in 1884 and includes a hospital for small animals, classrooms, and research facilities in the city. The large-animal hospital and research facilities are located at the New Bolton Center, an 800-acre farm 40 miles west of Philadelphia. The first 2 years are spent on the main campus. Part of the third year may be spent at the New Bolton Center, and the fourth year is spent in rotation and on electives at varying campus locations. Off-campus electives are frequently permitted.

Application Information

For specific application information (availability, deadlines, fees, and VMCAS participation), please refer to the contact information listed above.

Residency implications: priority is given to Pennsylvania residents. The number of nonresident places is usually about 80, including international applicants.

Prerequisites for Admission

At least 3 English credits must be in composition; biology courses must provide background in genetics and cell biology. Organic chemistry must cover aliphatic and aromatic compounds to fulfill the requirement.

Course requirements and semester hours

English (including composition)	6
Physics (with laboratory)	8
Chemistry (with at least 1 laboratory)	
General	8
Organic	4
Biology or zoology (covering the basics of genetics and cell bio)	9
Biochem (effective Fall 2014 entrance)	3
Microbiology (effective Fall 2014 entrance)	3
Social sciences or humanities	6
Calculus and math statistics (or biostats)	6
Electives	37

Required undergraduate GPA: no specific GPA. Applicants are evaluated comparatively. The mean cumulative GPA of the class admitted in 2012 was 3.59.

AP credit policy: must appear on official college transcripts and count toward degree.

Course completion deadline: prerequisite courses must be completed by the end of the summer term of the year in which admission is sought.

Standardized examinations: Graduate Record Examination (GRE®), general test, is required; the GRE Code for PennVet is 2775. Test scores should be received no later than December 1. The class admitted in 2012 had an average of 563 on the verbal subtest and 713 on the quantitative subtest.

Additional requirements and considerations

    Animal/veterinary work experience: experience working with animals, direct veterinary work, or research experience is desired. Approximately 500-600 hours is recommended. Experience should be sufficient to convince the admissions committee of motivation, interest, and understanding.

    Recommendations/evaluations: 3 required, one from an academic science source; and one from a veterinarian. The third is the choice of the applicant.

    Extracurricular/community service activities: additional activities in this category can provide information important to the admissions committee.

    Leadership: evidence of leadership abilities is desirable.

Summary of Admission Procedure

Timetable
> VMCAS application deadline: Wednesday, October 2, 2013 at 1:00 p.m.
> Eastern Time
> Supplemental application and fee deadline: October 2
> Date interviews are held: Fridays from early January until completion
> Date acceptances mailed: within 14 days after interview
> School begins: early September

Deposit (to hold place in class): $500.00. Deferments: are considered on an individual basis.

Evaluation criteria
The seats are filled through a 2-part admission procedure, which includes a file review and personal interviews.
> Grades
> Test scores
> Animal/veterinary experience
> Interview
> References
> Essay
> English skills (TOEFL)

File review: files are reviewed in January by pairs of members of the admissions committee (including an alumni member), and decisions are made on whether or not to offer an interview.

Personal interviews: interviews are held on Fridays from early January until the class is filled. The number of interviews granted equals 1½ to 2 times the number of seats available.

Two personal interviews are conducted: a formal interview with 2 faculty members (including an alumni member) of the committee, and an informal interview with student committee members. Although students do not vote on acceptance, they have a significant part in the meeting following interviews.

2011–2012 admissions summary for the class of 2016

	Number of Applicants	Number of New Entrants
Resident	200	12
Nonresident	1,193	83
Total:	1,393	125

Expenses for the 2012–2013 Academic Year

Tuition and fees
Resident	$37,304
Nonresident	$46,993

Dual-Degree Programs

Combined VMD–graduate degree programs are available.

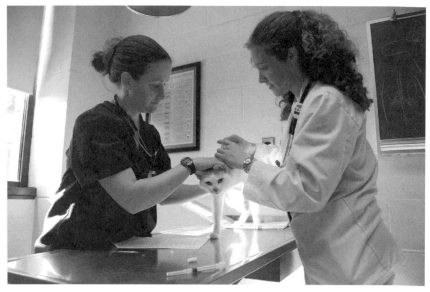

Fourth year students learning procedures at the Ryan Small Animal Hospital at the University of Pennsylvania School of Veterinary Medicine.

Purdue University

Student Services Center
Purdue University College of Veterinary Medicine
Lynn Hall, 1185
625 Harrison Street
West Lafayette, IN 47907-2026
Telephone: (765) 494-7893
Email: vetadmissions@purdue.edu
www.vet.purdue.edu

Purdue University is located in one of the largest metropolitan centers in northwestern Indiana. Greater Lafayette occupies a site on the Wabash River 65 miles northwest of Indianapolis and 126 miles southeast of Chicago. The combined population of the twin cities, Lafayette and West Lafayette, exceeds 100,000. The community offers an art museum, historical museum, 1,600 acres of public parks, and more than 60 churches of all major denominations.

Purdue ranks among the 25 largest colleges and universities in the nation. Students represent all 50 states and many foreign countries. Purdue University has the second highest enrollment of international students of any university in the United States. The Purdue University College of Veterinary Medicine strives to be the leading veterinary school for comprehensive education of the veterinary team and for discovery and engagement in selected areas of veterinary and comparative biomedical sciences. To better prepare individuals for veterinary medical careers in the twenty-first century, our curriculum emphasizes the veterinary team approach, problem-solving and hands-on experiences.

Application Information

For specific application information, please refer to the contact information listed above. Purdue Veterinary Medicine requires a brief supplemental application. The application can be obtained at www.vet.purdue.edu/admissions. The deadline for submission is October 2, 2013.

Each veterinary class has 84 students. The class will be seated with approximately 50% residents and 50% nonresident students.

Prerequisites for Admission

The course requirements outlined below are considered the minimum prerequisite courses to be completed. Grades no lower than C- must be received in each required course in order to be considered eligible for admission. In the electives category, humanities include languages, cognitive sciences, and social sciences. Other courses that are recommended to prepare you for the rigors of the professional program can be found on our web site.

Course requirements and number of semesters

Inorganic chemistry with lab	2
Organic chemistry with lab	2
Biochemistry	1
Biology with lab (diversity, developmental, cell structure)	2
Genetics with lab	1
Microbiology (general or medical) with lab	1
Nutrition (must be animal based)	1
Physics with lab	2
Calculus	1
Statistics	1
English composition	1
Communication (interpersonal, persuasion or speech)	1
Careers in Veterinary Medicine (if available)	1
Humanities (foreign languages, cognitive sciences, and social sciences)	3

Note: Complete course sequences should be followed rather than focusing on the number of semesters.

Required undergraduate GPA: the mean cumulative GPA of the entering class in the fall of 2012 was 3.59 on a 4.00 scale. The **minimum** cumulative GPA required for consideration is 2.75 on a 4.00.

AP credit policy: will be accepted if it appears on official college transcripts by subject area and is equivalent to the appropriate college-level coursework. Should your institution's official transcript not list the subject area, then you may submit an unofficial transcript with a letter from a university official explaining this and indicating which prerequisite courses are met by these credits.

Course completion deadline: minimum prerequisite courses must be completed by the end of the spring term prior to matriculation with the exception of Animal Nutrition which may be taken in the summer but must be completed prior to matriculation.

Standardized examinations: Graduate Record Examination (GRE®), general test, is required. **Test scores must be received no later than October 1 of the year of application.** As of 2013 application cycle, Purdue University will only accept scores of the revised GRE. Use the Grad School GRE code of 1631. There is no last date to complete the GRE.

Additional requirements and considerations
> Animal/veterinary/research experience
> Recommendations/evaluations (3 required; strongly suggested that one
> > reference is from a veterinarian)

Personal Statement
Employment record
Extracurricular college experience including leadership experience
Collegiate Honors and Awards

Summary of Admission Procedure

Timetable
> VMCAS application deadline: Wednesday, October 2, 2013 at 1:00 p.m.
> Eastern Time
> Purdue Supplemental Application deadline: October 1, 2013 at 1:00 p.m.
> Eastern Time
> Date interviews are held: January
> Date acceptances mailed: February
> Classes begin: late August

Deposit (to hold place in class): $250.00 for residents; $1,000.00 for non-residents. Deposit applied to tuition after matriculation.

Deferments: request for deferments will be considered on a case-by-case basis.

Evaluation criteria
The admission process consists of:
> A preliminary review based upon grade point indices, test scores, and prerequisite course completion
> An in-depth review of selected applicants
> A personal interview by invitation is required

	% weight
Grades, test scores, overall academic performance (including honors courses, study abroad)	55
Animal, veterinary, research, and general work experiences, extracurricular activities, personal statement, overall presentation of application materials, honors and awards, references, and interview	45

2012–2013 Applicant Summary

	Number of Applicants	Number of New Entrants
Resident	117	42
Nonresident	632	42
International	18	*
Total:	767	84

*International available seats are combined into non-resident number

Expenses for the 2012–2013 Academic Year

Tuition and fees
Resident	$19,326
Nonresident	$44,154

Dual-Degree Programs

Combined DVM-MS and DVM-PhD degree programs are available and tailored to suit the student's goals. Combined DVM-MPH degree program is available in cooperation with the University of Minnesota.

Early Admission Program

The Veterinary Scholars Program provides an opportunity for early admission into the professional program by accepting high-school seniors who have an outstanding high school academic record defined as:

1. rank in the top 10 percent of their graduating class or have a GPA > 3.50/4.00
2. have attained a combined SAT score $\geq$ 1930 or composite ACT score $\geq$ 28
3. strong science and mathematics background

Applicants must be admitted to Purdue University in a major of their choice. They must complete and submit the Veterinary Scholars application and all supporting materials by May 1st of the year in which they would begin their undergraduate program. Applicants are required to participate in personal interviews which are held on the Purdue campus, if invited.

Students admitted to the program must complete all preveterinary prerequisite coursework, and maintain stipulated cumulative grade point averages for each year of undergraduate study to remain in the program. Please see our website for more complete information: http://www.vet.purdue.edu/admissions/vet_scholars_webdocument.pdf

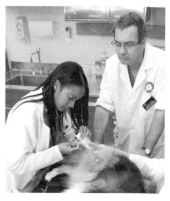

Purdue Veterinary Medicine offers significant clinical exposure where students develop excellent patient care, case management and client communication skills. Photo from: Mark Simons, Purdue News Service Photographer

University of Tennessee

Admissions Office
College of Veterinary Medicine
2407 River Drive
Room A-104-C
Knoxville TN 37996-4550
Telephone: (865) 974-7354
Email: dshepherd@utk.edu
www.vet.utk.edu

The University of Tennessee's College of Veterinary Medicine is located in Knoxville, a city of 185,000 situated in the Appalachian foothills of east Tennessee. Only 45 minutes from the Great Smoky Mountains National Park and 3 hours from both Nashville and Atlanta, Knoxville offers many recreational and cultural opportunities, including a symphony orchestra, an opera company, and several fine theaters. The climate in Knoxville is moderate with distinct seasons.

The 550-acre Knoxville campus of the University of Tennessee has about 21,300 undergraduate and 6,200 graduate students. The modern Clyde M. York Veterinary Medicine Building, housing the teaching and research facilities, the Veterinary Medical Center, including the W.W. Armistead Veterinary Teaching Hospitals (Equine, Farm Animal, Small Animal, and Avian, Exotic, and Zoological), and the Agriculture-Veterinary Medicine Library, faces the Tennessee River on the university's Agricultural Campus.

The curriculum of the College of Veterinary Medicine is a 9-semester, 4-year program. Development of a strong basic science education is emphasized in the first year. The second and third years emphasize the study of diseases, their causes, diagnosis, treatment, and prevention. Innovative features of the first three years of the curriculum include 6 weeks of student-centered small-group applied-learning exercises in semesters 1–5; 3 weeks of dedicated clinical experiences in the Veterinary Medical Center Hospitals in semesters 3–5; and elective course opportunities in semesters 4–9 that allow students to focus on specific educational/ career goals. In the fourth year (final 3 semesters), students participate exclusively in clinical rotations (29 weeks of core rotations and 15 weeks of elective rotations) in the Veterinary Medical Center and in required off-campus externships. The college has unique programs in zoo, avian, and exotic animal medicine and surgery, cancer diagnosis and therapy, minimally invasive surgery (laser lithotripsy, endoscopy, otoscopy), and rehabilitation/physical therapy.

Application Information

For specific application information (availability, deadlines, fees, and VMCAS participation), please refer to the contact information listed above. We admit approximately 85 applicants each year. Priority is given to Tennessee residents (60 of the 85 seats are for Tennessee residents). Twenty-five highly qualified non-residents are admitted each year.

Residency implications: Tennessee has no contractual agreements and does accept nonresident applications. Tennessee accepts applications only from United States citizens and permanent residents of the United States. International applications are not considered.

Prerequisites for Admission

Course requirements and semester hours

General inorganic chemistry (with laboratory)	8
Organic chemistry (with laboratory)	8
General biology/zoology (with laboratory)	8
Cellular/Molecular biology*	3
Genetics	3
Biochemistry (exclusive of laboratory)†	4
Physics (with laboratory)	8
English composition	6
Social sciences/humanities	18

* It is expected that this requirement will be fulfilled by a course in cellular or molecular biology. An upper-division cell or molecular biology course is preferred.

† This should be a complete upper-division course in general cellular and comparative biochemistry. Half of a 2-semester sequence will not satisfy this requirement.

Applicants are strongly encouraged to complete additional biological and physical science courses, especially comparative anatomy, mammalian physiology, microbiology with laboratory, and statistics.

AP credit policy: must appear on official college transcripts and be equivalent to the appropriate college-level coursework.

Required undergraduate GPA: for nonresident applicants, the minimum acceptable cumulative GPA is 3.20 on a 4.00 scale. At time of acceptance, the mean GPA of the class entering in fall of 2012 was 3.53.

Course completion deadline: prerequisite courses must be completed with a grade of C or better by the end of the spring term prior to entry.

Standardized examinations: Graduate Record Exam (GRE®), General Test (Verbal, Quantitative, and Analytical) is required, and scores must be received by November 15, 2013. The last date applicants should plan on taking the GRE is October 1, 2013. UTK's GRE code is 2104, and the Department Code is 0617. For applicants planning to matriculate in August, 2014, results of GRE tests taken prior to November 1, 2009, will not be accepted.

Additional requirements and considerations
> Animal/veterinary work experience
> 3 letters of recommendation are required and preferred. No more than 5 letters will be accepted
> Extracurricular and/or community service activities
> Leadership skills
> Autobiographical essay (personal statement)
> A Supplemental Application is required and can be found at: http://www.utk.edu/admissions/supplemental.php.

Summary of Admission Procedure

Timetable
> VMCAS application deadline: Wednesday, October 2, 2013 at 1:00 p.m. Eastern Time
> GRE Scores must be received by the College no later than November 15, 2013
> Date interviews are held: March 17-21, 2014
> Date acceptances mailed: no later than April 1
> Applicant's response date: April 15
> School begins: late August

Deposit (to hold place in class): none required. Deferments: are considered on a case-by-case basis.

Evaluation criteria
The admission procedure consists of an initial file review followed by an interview of selected applicants.
> Initial academic file review:
>> Grades
>> Test scores
>> VMCAS and Supplemental Application information
> Interview
>> Animal/veterinary experience
>> Evidence of logical preparation for this career
>> Extracurricular activities/community service
>> Personal interests and qualities
>> References (3-5 required)
>> Personal Statement

2012–2013 admissions summary

	Number of Applicants	Number of New Entrants
Resident	127	64
Nonresident	538	24
Total:	665	88

Expenses for the 2012–2013 Academic Year

Tuition and fees
Resident	$22,616
Nonresident	$49,142

Parallel Degree Program

The College, in partnership with the College of Education, Health and Human Sciences, offers an option for veterinary students (and graduate veterinarians) to earn the MPH degree with a concentration in Veterinary Public Health. Contact the College of Veterinary Medicine, Dr. John Coy New Jr. at jnew@utk.edu for additional information.

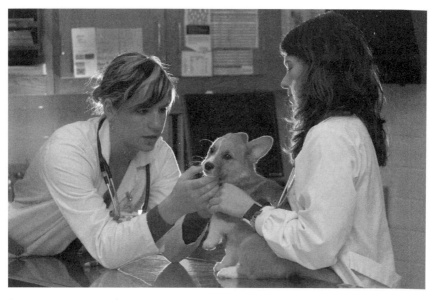

Senior veterinary students examine a patient in the Small Animal Teaching Hospital of the University of Tennessee Veterinary Medical Center.

Texas A & M University

Office of the Dean
Attn: Student Admissions
College of Veterinary Medicine & Biomedical Sciences
Texas A & M University
College Station TX 77843-4461
Telephone: (979) 862-1169
vetmed.tamu.edu

The university is located adjacent to the cities of Bryan and College Station. The two cities have a combined population of about 100,000. The student population at Texas A & M is more than 40,000. The College of Veterinary Medicine is one of the 10 original veterinary teaching institutions that existed in the United States prior to World War II.

The College provides an integrated professional curriculum that prepares graduates with a firm foundation in the basic sciences, a broad comparative medicine knowledge base, and the clinical and personal skills to be leaders in the many career fields of veterinary medicine. Professional students are given the opportunity to gain additional education and training in their personal career paths.

Becoming a veterinarian requires much dedication and diligent study. The veterinary medical student is required to meet a high level of performance. The demands on students' time and effort are considerable, but the rewards and career satisfaction are personal achievements that make significant contributions to our society.

Application Information

For specific application information (availability, deadlines and fees), please refer to the contact information listed above.

Residency implications: Texas has no contractual agreements with other states. Applicants from other states who have outstanding credentials will be considered. Texas seats 122 residents and up to 10 non-resident applicants per year. In the event that not all 10 non-resident positions are filled, these positions will then be filled with Texas alternates. Successful candidates who are awarded competitive university-based scholarships may attend at resident tuition rate.

Prerequisites for Admission

The minimum number of college or university credits required for admission into the professional curriculum is 62 semester hours. Applicants must have completed or have in progress approximately 46 credit hours at the time of application. Because there is no specific degree plan associated with pre-veterinary education, students are encouraged to pursue a degree plan that meets individual interests. Students are strongly encouraged to choose courses with the assistance of a knowledgeable counselor at the undergraduate institution or through contact with an academic advisor at the College of Veterinary Medicine, telephone: (979) 862-1169.

Course requirements and semester hours (subject to change)

Life sciences

General biology (with laboratory)	4
General microbiology (with laboratory)	4
*Genetics	3
*Animal nutrition or feeds and feeding	3

Chemical-physical sciences and mathematics

Inorganic chemistry (with laboratory)	8
Organic chemistry (with laboratory)	8
*Biochemistry I & II(lecture hours only)	5
*Statistics	3
Physics (with laboratory)	8

Nonscience

Composition and Rhetoric	3
General Psychology course	3
Speech Communications	3
Technical writing	3

* These courses must be taken at a 4-year college or university. These courses may not be taken at community or junior colleges.

Required undergraduate GPA: the minimum overall GPA required is 2.90 on a 4.00 scale or 3.10 for the last 45 semester credits. The mean of the most recent entering class was 3.65.

AP credit policy: AP credit is accepted as fulfilling selected prerequisites; credit must be reflected on the official undergraduate transcript.

Course completion deadline: required courses must be completed by the end of the spring term prior to entry.

Standardized examinations: Graduate Record Examination (GRE®), general test, is required. Beginning August 1, 2011, the College of Veterinary Medicine will require the new version of the GRE examination only. Any exam taken prior to this date will not be accepted. The last date to take the GRE (general test) exam is September 30 of the year of application.

Additional requirements and considerations
    Evaluations
    Animal/veterinary work experience

Animal and veterinary experience is considered to evaluate the applicant's personal qualities and motivation to be a veterinarian.

Animal experience includes caring for and handling animals in a kennel or animal shelter. It also includes any other experience that was not under the direct supervision of a veterinarian, such as FFA and 4-H projects. Veterinary experience is hours spent working under the direct supervisions of a veterinarian, whether in a clinical or research environment, paid or volunteer. **Applicants must have more than 50 hours' worth of veterinary experience in order to qualify for an interview.**

Points are assigned based on the number of hours worked and the variety of environments in which the hours were obtained. These two experiences are scored separately, so applicants should obtain experience in both areas. For example, an applicant who worked for a veterinarian should include time spent cleaning stalls or cages as animal experience and time spent with the veterinarian as veterinary experience.

Summary of Admission Procedure

Timetable
    Application deadline: October 1
    Date interviews are held: mid-January
    Date acceptances mailed: mid-March
    School begins: late August

Deposit (to hold place in class): none required.

Deferments: requests for deferments will be considered on a case-by-case basis.

Evaluation criteria
    Academic performance
    Test scores
    Interview
    Personal statement
    Evaluations (3 evaluations are required. 1 evaluation must come from a veterinarian with whom you have worked. Failure to complete this request could result in the disqualification of your application. No additional letters of support/recommendation are needed.)
    Semester course load and postacademic challenge
    Leadership and experience

2011–2012 admissions summary

	Number of Applicants	Number of New Entrants
Resident	353	125
Nonresident	<u>116</u>	<u>8</u>
Total:	469	133

Expenses for the 2011–2012 Academic Year

Tuition and fees
Resident	$20,478
Nonresident	$31,278

Tufts University

Office of Admissions
Cummings School of Veterinary Medicine
Tufts University
200 Westboro Road
North Grafton MA 01536
Telephone: (508) 839-7920
Email: vetadmissions@tufts.edu
www.tufts.edu/vet/

Tufts University is located near Boston, where athletic and cultural activities abound. The Cummings School of Veterinary Medicine provides an exciting biomedical environment for the study of modern veterinary medicine. Signature opportunities include Wildlife and Conservation Medicine, International Veterinary Medicine, Accelerated Clinical Excellence, and Animal Welfare, Ethics, and Policy. Hands-on learning begins in the first year and continues throughout the next three years. Many opportunities exist outside of formal courses for hands-on work in hospitals and research laboratories. The Hospital for Large Animals, Foster Hospital for Small Animals, the Ambulatory Service, and the Wildlife Clinic provide a rich mixture of horses, cats, dogs, cattle, sheep, goats, and native wildlife. Our large caseload, typically ranked among the top three schools in the country, provides exciting learning opportunities for students.

Application Information

For specific application information (availability, deadlines, fees, and VMCAS participation), please refer to the contact information listed above.

Residency implications: Massachusetts residents make up about one-third of each class. All others considered for the remaining spaces.

Prerequisites for Admission

Course requirements and semesters

Biology (with laboratory)	2
Inorganic chemistry (with laboratory)	2
Organic chemistry (with laboratory)	2
Physics	2
Mathematics	2
Genetics, unless included in biology	1
Biochemistry	1
English composition	2

| Social and behavioral sciences | 2 |
| Humanities and fine arts | 2 |

Required undergraduate GPA: no minimum GPA required. The average GPA for the class admitted in 2012 was 3.64.

AP credit policy: must appear on official college transcripts and be equivalent to the appropriate college-level coursework.

Course completion deadline: prerequisite courses must be completed by the time of matriculation into the DVM program.

Standardized examinations: Graduate Record Examinations (GRE®), general test, is required. The most recent acceptable test date for applicants to the class of 2018 is October 31, 2013. The oldest acceptable scores must be within 5 years of the application deadline. Average GRE scores for the class of 2016 were verbal 160, quantitative 158, and analytical 4.5.

Additional requirements and considerations
    Animal/veterinary/biomedical research/health science experience
    Rigor of coursework
    Knowledge of the profession
    Letters of Evaluation (3 required)
       advisor/faculty members
       veterinarian/research scientist
    Essays
    Interview
    Extracurricular /community service activities
    Leadership potential

Summary of Admission Procedure

Timetable
    Application deadline: November 1
    Date interviews are held: December, January, February
    Date acceptances mailed: March
    School begins: late August

Deposit (to hold place in class): $500.00.

Deferments: requests for deferment are handled on a case-by-case basis.

Evaluation criteria
Tufts' admission procedure consists of a review of the application and an interview of selected applicants.

2012–2013 admissions summary

	Number of Applicants	*Number of New Entrants*
Total:	766	96

Expenses for the 2011–2012 Academic Year

Tuition and fees
Resident $41,062
Nonresident $44,346

Dual-Degree Program

Combined DVM–graduate degree programs are available.

International applicants are considered for admission.

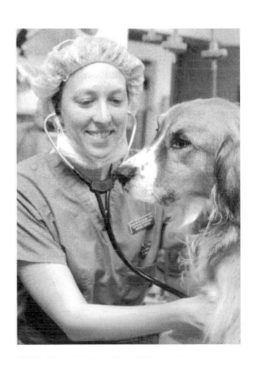

Veterinary medical students find their clinical rounds not only educational but also personally satisfying. Photo courtesy of Tufts University Cummings School of Veterinary Medicine.

Tuskegee University

Office of Veterinary Admissions and Recruitment Tuskegee University School of Veterinary Medicine, Tuskegee, AL 36088
Telephone: (334) 727-8460
Website: www.onemedicine.tuskegee.edu

Tuskegee University School of Veterinary Medicine is located in Tuskegee, Alabama, a city of about 13,000. Tuskegee is 40 miles east of the state of Alabama, Capitol city, Montgomery, and twenty miles west of the city of Auburn. It is also within easy driving distance to the cities of Birmingham, Alabama and Atlanta, Georgia. Summers are hot with moderate to mild humidity, and winters are moderate. Its recreational facilities, lakes, and parks can be enjoyed throughout the year-round.

Over the past 125 years and still today, since it was founded by Booker T. Washington in 1881, Tuskegee University (HBCU) has become one of our nation's most outstanding institutions of higher learning. While it focuses on helping to develop human resources primarily within the African-American community, it is open to all.

Tuskegee's mission has always been to provide service to people in addition to education. The University stresses the need to educate the whole person, that is, the hand and the heart as well as the mind. Tuskegee enrolls more than 3,000 students and employs approximately 900 faculty and support personnel. Physical facilities include more than 5,000 acres of forestry and a campus consisting of more than 100 major buildings and structures. Total land, forestry, and facilities are valued in excess of $500 million. The campus has also been declared a historical site by the United States Department of the Interior.

Historically, Tuskegee University School of Veterinary Medicine (TUSVM) was established in 1945 for the training of African-Americans during a time when few had the opportunity to study veterinary medicine because of segregation and other racial impediments.

In 1945, the United States had only 10 schools of veterinary medicine and it is estimated that fewer than five African Americans were located in the southern states. TUSVM graduated its first class of fully qualified veterinarians in 1949. Since then, it has graduated more than 70% of the African-American veterinarians in the United States.

Today, TUSVM is one of 28 Schools/Colleges of Veterinary Medicine in the United States. However, it is the only one in the U.S. that is fully integrated, serving African-Americans, Caucasian students, Hispanics, Asians, Native Americans and international students. TUSVM is the most racially, 125 ethnically, and culturally diverse school of veterinary medicine in North America.

Also, TUSVM's graduates have excelled in private clinical practice, in public practice such as in the government, in the military, and in corporations such as the pharmaceutical industry. They hold key leadership positions in the government, military, academia, and in the international arena.

Tuskegee University School of Veterinary Medicine is fully accredited by the American Veterinary Medical Association (AVMA) and its Veterinary Teaching Hospital is accredited by the American Animal Hospital Association (AAHA).

Application Information

Application Fee: $205.00 TUSVM requires a processing fee to develop and maintain each applicant's computerized database. Send Application fee directly to Tuskegee University School of Veterinary Medicine-Office of Admissions and Recruitment.

For specific application information (availability, deadlines, fees, and VM-CAS), please refer to the contact information listed above, or visit the online application process at: www.onemedicine.tuskegee.edu.

Residency implications: applications are accepted with special consideration given to Alabama residents and those who have residency in the following contract states, Kentucky, South Carolina, and Arkansas.

Number of resident seats, non-resident seat: none - TUSVM maintains "open access" and selection for seats.

International applications will be considered for admissions into TUSVM

Prerequisites for Admission

The Tuskegee University School of Veterinary Medicine's professional curriculum is a rigorous four-year program. Therefore applicant's final grade for each required course must be a "C" or better. Students are required to take the General Aptitude portion of the Graduate Record Examination (GRE). Additionally, there is a mandatory interview with the TUSVM Admissions Committee before acceptance into the school is granted.

GPA: the cumulative and science GPA requirement is 2.7 on a 4.00 scale.

Course completion deadline: prerequisite courses must be completed by end of May.

Standardized examinations: Graduate Record Examination (GRE) of which must be taken within three years of application, is required. Must be completed by October 1. Request GRE Test Scores results by November 1.

Courses and Requirements in Semester Hours

I. English or Written Composition	6
II. Mathematics	6
III. Social Sciences / Humanities	6
IV. Liberal Arts	<u>6</u>
	24

VI. Biological & Physical Sciences

Advance Biology (300 Level or Above)**	9
Biochemistry w/Lab	4
Advance Biology Elective	8
Organic Chemistry w/Lab	4
Physics w/Lab	<u>8</u>
	33

VI. Animal Science***

Introduction to Animal Science	3
Animal Nutrition	<u>3</u>
	6

Total Semester Hours 63

** Advanced biology courses, e.g., anatomy, physiology, ecology, immunology, zoology, microbiology, genetics, toxicology, and histology

*** Applicants who do not include animal science courses in their Pre-Professional studies may be admitted at the discretion of the Admissions Committee, if they fulfilled all other requirements. However, these courses must be completed prior to attaining third-year status in the Tuskegee University School of Veterinary Medicine. From year 2017 forward all animal science courses have to be completed before enrollment at the veterinary school.

Summary of Admission Procedure

Timetable

Application deadline: October 1
Date interviews are held: January–February
Date acceptances mailed: April 15
School begins: mid-August

Deferments: one-year deferments are considered on a case-by-case basis.

Evaluation criteria

The following items are taken into consideration: academic record, academic trends, letters of recommendation, work experience, and test scores.

	% weight
Grades	68
Test scores	8
Animal/veterinary experience	6
Interview	15

References
    Science Professors   2
    Veterinarian   1
    Essay (Handwritten, see application)

Number of available seats - Approximately 65-70

Expenses for the 2012–2013 Academic Year

Tuition and fees
    In state $10,860.00 per semester
    Out of state $18,135.00 per semester
    Technology fee $200.00
    I.D. fee $30.00
    Application Fee: $205.00
    If admitted, additional fees and expenses are required.

Dual-Degree Programs

Combined DVM–Graduate Degree Programs are available: PhD in Integrative
Biosciences, PhD Interdisciplinary Pathobiology, Master of Science Veterinary
Science, Master of Science Tropical Animal Health, Master of Public Health
and Master of Science in Public Health

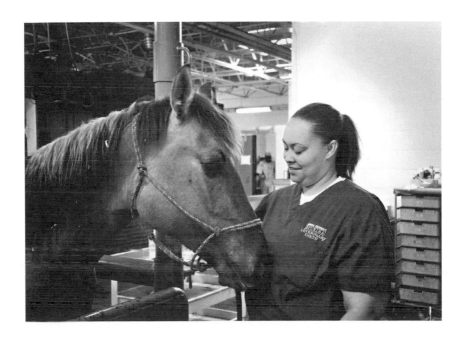

Virginia-Maryland Regional College of Veterinary Medicine

Admissions Coordinator
Virginia-Maryland Regional College of Veterinary Medicine
Blacksburg VA 24061
Telephone: (540) 231-4699
Fax: (540) 231-9290
Email: dvmadmit@vt.edu
http://www.becomeavet.vetmed.vt.edu/

The Virginia-Maryland Regional College of Veterinary Medicine is situated on 3 distinct campuses. The main campus is at Virginia Tech in Blacksburg, Virginia, a community with a population of about 40,000 situated on a high plateau in southwestern Virginia between the Blue Ridge and Allegheny Mountains. Its residents enjoy a wide range of educational, social, recreational, and cultural opportunities. In addition to the Blacksburg campus, the Equine Medical Center campus is in Leesburg, Virginia, and the University of Maryland is at College Park.

In recognition of a need for veterinarians trained in both basic and clinical sciences, the college offers students the opportunity to participate in graduate studies and receive appropriate advanced training to conduct research in basic or clinical disciplines. Nearly 25 percent of the nation's veterinarians work in areas other than private practice, such as government and corporate veterinary medicine. Through the assistance of a grant from the Pew Charitable Trusts, the college has established the Center for Public and Corporate Veterinary Medicine, which is a national resource for training veterinarians for the wide variety of careers in this area of the profession.

Application Information

For specific application information (availability, deadlines, fees, and VMCAS participation), please refer to the contact information listed above.

Residency implications: 50 positions are reserved for Virginia residents, and 30 positions for Maryland residents. Up to 40 additional positions may be filled by nonresidents, 6 of those reserved for WV residents.

Prerequisites for Admission

Course requirements and semester hours
Biological sciences (with laboratories)	8
Organic chemistry (with laboratories)	8

Physics (with laboratories)	8
Biochemistry	3
English (composition, 3 credit hours)	6
Humanities/social science	6
Mathematics (algebra, geometry, trigonometry, calculus)	6

Students must earn a C– or better in all required courses.

Science courses taken 7 or more years ago may be repeated or substituted with higher-level courses with the written consent of the admissions committee.

Required undergraduate GPA: to be considered for admission, applicants must have a cumulative GPA of at least 2.80 on a 4.00 scale upon completion of a minimum of 2 academic years of full-time study (60 semester/90 quarter hours) at an accredited college or university. Alternatively, a 3.30 GPA in the last 2 years (60 semester hours) will qualify a student who does not have a 2.80 GPA overall. All courses taken during this 2-year period must be junior or senior level. The mean GPA of those accepted into the class of 2016 was 3.5.

Advanced placement credit for 1 semester of English will be accepted if the additional required hours are composition or technical writing and are taken at a college or university.

Advanced placement credit or credit by examination for the other preveterinary course requirements will be accepted. Those credits must appear on the applicant's college transcript. Advanced placement credits will not be calculated in grade point averages and no grade assigned. No course substitutions will be allowed for AP credit or credit by examination.

Course completion deadline: required courses must be completed by the end of the spring term of the year in which matriculation occurs.

Standardized examinations: Graduate Record Examination (GRE®) scores must be received by November 1, 2013. It is advised that the test be taken by the first week of October.

Letters of recommendation: Three electronic evaluations/letters of recommendation are required.

Additional requirements and considerations
    Maturity and a broad cultural perspective
    Motivation and dedication to a career in veterinary medicine

Evidence of potential, and appreciation of the career opportunities for veterinarians, as indicated by:

1. Clinical veterinary experience (private practice)
2. Animal experience in addition to time spent working with a veterinarian
3. Biomedical/research experience (such as working with veterinarians or other biomedically trained individuals in health care, government, research laboratories, industrial, or corporate settings.)
4. Extramural activities, achievements, honors
5. Communication skills
6. References

Summary of Admission Procedure

Timetable
> VMCAS application deadline: Wednesday, October 2, 2013 at 1:00 p.m. Eastern Time
> Supplemental application deadline: October 2, 2013 (The supplemental application can be accessed at: https://banweb.banner.vt.edu/ssb/prod/hzskvmga.P_VetMed
> Date interviews are held: TBD
> Date acceptances mailed: early March
> School begins: mid-August

Deposit (to hold place in class): $450.00 for Maryland and Virginia residents; $1,000.00 for nonresidents.

Deferments: case-by-case basis if a candidate has extenuating circumstances beyond his or her control.

Evaluation criteria
The admission procedure is comprised of an initial screening of applicants, review of the application portfolios, and interviews of selected applicants.

Evaluation
> 70% - Academics: cumulative GPA, required science GPA, last 45 semester hour GPA, GRE aptitude
> 30% - Non-Academics: related animal experience, veterinary experience; research, industrial, and biomedical experiences; references; and overall application portfolio review

Interviews
Top candidates ranked on the above criteria will be invited for interviews. Admission offers will be based on interview results.

2012–2013 admissions summary

	Number of Applicants	Number of New Entrants
Resident		
Maryland	127	30
Virginia	182	50
Nonresident	826	40
Total:	1,135	120

Expenses for the 2012–2013 Academic Year

Tuition and fees

Resident	$21,434
Nonresident	$46,366

Dual-Degree Programs

Combined DVM–graduate degree programs are available.

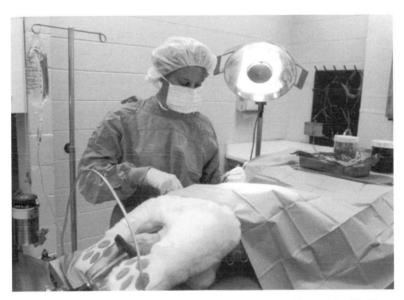

A junior veterinary student practices suturing techniques during the "Teddy Bear Repair Clinic" at the Virginia-Maryland Regional College of Veterinary Medicine's annual Open House. Photo courtesy of Biomedical Media Center, VMRCVM.

Washington State University

Office of Student Services
College of Veterinary Medicine
Washington State University
P. O. Box 647012
Pullman WA 99164-7012
Telephone: (509) 335-1532
Email: admissions@vetmed.wsu.edu
Website: www.vetmed.wsu.edu

Washington-Idaho-Utah (WIU) Regional Program in Veterinary Medicine is located in Pullman in southeastern Washington. The 60,000 people who live in the communities of Pullman, WA, and Moscow, ID, live and study here because the area has much to offer those who seek a lifestyle that combines a beautiful country setting with the benefits of two major universities (University of Idaho is just a few miles away in Moscow, ID). Plus, WSU is a member of the PAC-12 athletic conference so exciting sporting events are never short on supply. With a true four season climate, beautiful rivers, and nearby mountains, there are excellent recreational activities available ranging from hiking, mountain biking, skiing and snowboarding, to fishing, camping and whitewater rafting.

The College of Veterinary Medicine was founded in 1899 and is one of the oldest colleges of veterinary medicine in the country. Seven major buildings house the Departments of Veterinary Clinical Sciences, Comparative Anatomy Pharmacology and Physiology, and Microbiology and Pathology, along with the Washington Animal Disease Diagnostic Laboratory, the School for Molecular Biosciences, and the Paul G. Allen School for Global Animal Health. The faculty and staff of the Veterinary Teaching Hospital are considered leaders in the field of veterinary diagnostic imaging. The well regarded oncology unit offers an active clinical service delivering medical and radiation oncology to a wide variety of companion animals. The hospital attracts a large and diverse caseload for the DVM educational program. The veterinary teaching program also allows for students to take advantage of numerous off-campus clinical opportunities in all areas of veterinary medicine.

The college is a leader in the development of programs to promote and enhance emotional intelligence, leadership and communication skills. The School for Global Animal Health, the first of its kind in North America, is serving as the centerpiece of the college's expanded research on animal diseases that directly impact human health. For those DVM students interested in gaining research experience, numerous opportunities exist, including the competitive Research Scholars Program, which is designed to encourage the exploration of research careers in veterinary medicine.

Washington State University College of Veterinary Medicine (WSU CVM) has long been partners with the state of Idaho and the Western Interstate Commission of Higher Education (WICHE) program.

A new educational partnership with Utah State University was established in March of 2011. Students selected into the Utah track within the WIU program will spend their first two years in Logan, Utah where much of the curriculum will be taught by the faculty of USU's Department of Animal, Dairy and Veterinary Sciences (ADVS), paralleling the curriculum taught in Pullman. USU boasts internationally recognized faculty members, cutting edge technology, and excellent animal and research facilities. Parts of the first two years will be taught by Pullman-based faculty, and the final two years are completed at the WSU CVM in Pullman, WA.

The regional program allows students the unique educational opportunity to experience world class education from two distinguished universities. The Utah track will accept 20 Utah resident applicants and up to 10 non-resident applicants per year.

Application Information

For the most current application information (availability, deadlines, fees, and VMCAS participation), please refer to the contact information listed above.

Residency implications: In general, first preference is given to qualified applicants who are residents of Washington, Idaho and Utah, as well as qualified applicants certified by WICHE contract states. Second preference is given to qualified applicants from non-service area states and non-certified or non-sponsored applicants from WICHE states.

At the Pullman site there are up to (60) available seats for Washington residents, (11) Idaho residents, and up to (25) non-residents.

At the Logan site there will be (20) Utah residents and 10 non-residents.

There are two programs at Washington State University by which highly motivated and uniquely qualified individuals may gain early acceptance (pre-admission) and early entry (admission) into the professional veterinary medical program. In cooperation with the WSU College of Veterinary Medicine, the University Honors College offers the Pre-Admitted Veterinary Medicine Program and the Department of Animal Sciences offers the Combined Program in Animal Science and Veterinary Medicine. These programs are available only to WSU undergraduate students.

Prerequisites for Admission

Course requirements and semester hours

Biology (with lab)	8
Inorganic Chemistry (with lab)	8
Organic Chemistry (with lab)	4
Physics (with lab)	4
Math (precalculus or higher)	3
Genetics	4
Biochemistry	3
Statistical Methods	3
Arts/Humanities/Social Sciences/History*	21
English Composition/Communication*	6
Total	64

These requirements will be waived if a student has a bachelor's degree.

Required undergraduate GPA: none; a minimum overall GPA of 3.20 on a 4.00 scale is recommended.

AP credit policy: Must meet Washington State University requirements.

Course completion deadline: Prerequisite courses must be completed before time of matriculation.

Standardized examinations: Graduate Record Examination (GRE®), general test, is required. Test scores older than 5 years will not be accepted. Test scores are due by October 1, 2013. Applicants are encouraged to take the exam by August 1, 2013.

Additional requirements and considerations

Animal/veterinary/research/work experience
Letters of Recommendation (LOR) (An academic and veterinary LOR are both required)
Extracurricular and/or community service activities
Personal Statement
Supplemental Application

Summary of Admission Procedure

Timetable
> VMCAS application deadline: Wednesday, October 2, 2013 at 1:00 p.m. Eastern Time; WSU Supplemental: Tuesday, October 8, 2013 by 5 p.m. PST (The supplemental application can be accessed at http://www.vetmed.wsu.edu/prospectiveStudents/)
> Date interviews are held: January–February
> Date acceptances mailed: January–April
> School begins: late August

Deposit (to hold place in class): None required.

Deferments: Considered on a case-by-case basis.

Evaluation criteria
Applicants will be selected based upon ability to successfully complete the program and demonstration of the qualities that make a successful veterinarian. Academic criteria include grades, quality and rigor of academic program and GRE test scores. Non-academic factors include animal/veterinary/research/work experience, honors & awards, community service, extracurricular activities, essay, letters of recommendation; other factors include maturity, integrity, compassion, communication skills, and desire to contribute to society. An interview is required for Washington and Idaho residents, as well as for out-of-area, non-resident applicants. WICHE applicants are ranked for WICHE funding using the same criteria above minus the interview.

2012 Admissions Summary

	Number of Applicants	Number of New Entrants
Washington	151	50
Idaho	43	12
Utah	43	21
WICHE†	182	30
Nonresident	633	13
Total:	1,052	126

† For further information, see the listing of contracting states and provinces.

Expenses for the 2012–2013 Academic Year

Tuition and fees - WSU Pullman, WA Site
    Resident (WA, ID, and WICHE supported) $21,830
    Nonresident $52,854

Tuition and fees - WSU Logan, UT Site
    Resident $22,378
    Nonresident with scholarship $45,422
    Nonresident without scholarship $53,422

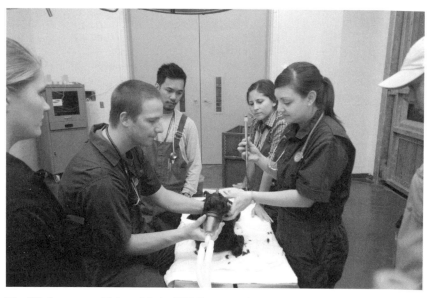

The Washington – Idaho – Utah (WIU) Regional Program in veterinary medicine offers DVM students hands-on experience starting year one.

Western University of Health Sciences

Office of Admission
College of Veterinary Medicine
Western University of Health Sciences
309 East 2nd Street
Pomona, CA 91766-1854
Phone: (909) 623-6116 FAX: (909) 469-5570
E-mail: admissions@westernu.edu
Web site: http://www.prospective.westernu.edu/veterinary/requirements
Link to Application: https://banapps.westernu.edu:4443/pls/live8/bwskalog.P_
DispLoginNon

Western University of Health Sciences is an independent, accredited, non-profit university incorporated in the State of California, dedicated to educating compassionate and competent health professionals who value diversity and a humanistic approach to patient care. The university, located in the San Gabriel Valley of Southern California, about 30 miles east of Los Angeles, grants post baccalaureate professional degrees in nine colleges: the College of Podiatric Medicine, the College of Dental Medicine, the College of Optometry, the Graduate College of Biomedical Sciences, the College of Allied Health Professions, the College of Graduate Nursing, the College of Osteopathic Medicine of the Pacific, the College of Pharmacy, and the College of Veterinary Medicine. The American Veterinary Medical Association Council on Education granted the College of Veterinary Medicine full accreditation status in 2010. Western U's CVM admitted its charter class Fall 2003. The founding principles of the College of Veterinary Medicine include:

1) *Commitment to student-centered, life-long learning.*
   The curriculum is designed to teach students to find and critically evaluate information, to enhance student cooperative learning, and to provide an environment for professional development.

2) *Commitment to a Reverence for Life philosophy in teaching veterinary medicine.*
   The College strives to make the educational experience one that enhances moral development of its students and is respectful to all animals and people involved in its programs. Students only practice clinical and surgical skills on live animals when it is medically necessary for that animal.

3) *Commitment to excellence of student education through strategic partnerships in the public and private veterinary sectors.*
   This commitment seeks to maximize the learning experience in veterinary clinical practice and to educate practice-ready veterinarians capable of functioning independently upon graduation. In the 3rd & 4th years of the curriculum students are trained primarily off-campus at state of the art facilities.

Curriculum

The first two years of the four-year curriculum provide education in basic and clinical veterinary science using a small-group, problem-based learning format, a Veterinary Issues course, a Molecular Biology course, and a Clinical Skills course. These courses rely on learning environments such as the on-campus Multi-disciplinary laboratory, Thing Lab, and Banfield Veterinary Clinical Center, and the off-campus Companion Animal Wellness clinic, Large animal wellness, California State Polytechnic University-Pomona, and off-campus ambulatory programs. Years three and four are comprised of clinical rotations at participating veterinary practices and biomedical learning environments.

Phase I (Years 1 & 2): Basic and clinical veterinary science education using problem-based learning modules, a veterinary issues seminar series, a molecular biology seminar series, and an experiential clinical skills course.

Phase II (Year 3): Required rotations in thirteen different areas of veterinary medicine in regional veterinary practices or institutions including some rotations conducted on campus.

Phase III (Year 4): Selective rotations in regional, national or international specialty practices, veterinary teaching hospitals, or public/private institutions to be determined by students' career goals.

Application Information

For specific application information (availability, deadlines, fees, and VMCAS participation), please refer to the contact information listed previously.

Residency implications: applicants from all states as well as international applicants will be considered. In-state and out-of-state applicants are given equal consideration.

Prerequisites for Admissions

Course requirements[1]:

	Semester Units	Quarter Units
Organic chemistry (including laboratory)	3	4
Biochemistry or Physiological Chemistry[2,3]	3	4
Biological & Life Sciences[3,4,5] (must be upper-division Biological & Life Sciences and include one upper-division laboratory course)*	9	12
Microbiology[3,5]	3	4
Physiology[3,5]	3	4
Genetics or Molecular Biology[3,5]	3	4

General physics (including laboratory)	6	8
Statistics[2]	3	4
English composition	6	8
Public Speaking or Small Group Communication	3	4
Humanities/social sciences/ psychology/sociology	9	12

* Ex: biology, physiology, anatomy, cell biology, embryology, zoology, immunology

1,2,3,4,5: See Course completion deadline on following page for details.

Required undergraduate GPA: Applicants must have a minimum overall, prerequisite science, and prerequisite GPA of 2.75 (undergraduate and graduate) at the time of application to be considered for admission. The minimum GPAs must be maintained through matriculation into the program. Prerequisite courses must be completed with a grade of C (or its equivalent) or higher.

AP credit policy: must appear on official college transcripts and be equivalent to the appropriate college-level coursework. AP test subject and number of credits must also be specified on the transcript.

Course completion deadline: (1) All courses must be completed at a regionally accredited college or university in the United States. Exceptions will be made on a case-by-case basis. Coursework completed outside the U.S. (including Canada) must be evaluated by a WesternU approved evaluation service (please visit the requirements page of the website for a listing of approved services). All required courses must be completed by the end of the spring term of planned matriculation year. Failure to satisfactorily complete prerequisites with a grade of C or better will result in the loss of a candidate's seat in the class. One course cannot be used to satisfy more than one prerequisite. (2) Must be a course designed or specified for science majors. (3) These required courses must have been completed no more than 8 years prior to the date of matriculation at WesternU-CVM. Classes taken after August 1, 2006, will be considered within the 8-year time limit and may be applied toward the prerequisites for the class entering Fall 2014. (4) While not specifically required, courses in anatomy, nutrition, immunology, and embryology are strongly encouraged. (5) All except two of these courses must be completed by the end of the Fall term immediately prior to the planned year of matriculation at WesternU-CVM.

Standardized examinations: Graduate Record Examination (GRE®), general test, or Medical College Admissions Test (MCAT) is required. Test scores must be received by the October 15, 2013, supplemental application deadline. Test scores older than five years prior to the planned year of matriculation are not acceptable.

Additional requirements and considerations:

Animal experience: must total at least 500 hours of hands-on experience that goes beyond observation. Appropriate venues include but are not limited to: animal medical environment/ veterinary practice; commercial animal production; regulatory animal control; animal entertainment or research environment.

Recommendations/evaluations: 3 are required from among the following: previous employers, supervisors of extended volunteer activities, academic personnel.

Interview

Summary of Admissions Procedure

Timetable

VMCAS application deadline: Wednesday, October 2, 2013 at 1:00 p.m. Eastern Time

Supplemental application deadline: electronically submitted with the prerequisite worksheet on or before October 15, 2013 at 11:59 PDT

Date interviews are held: January–February

Date acceptances mailed: March

School begins: August

Deposit (to hold place in class): $500.

Deferments: request for deferments will be considered on a case-by-case basis.

Evaluation criteria:

Academic achievement

Standardized test performance

Animal experience

Letters of reference

Interview

Other supporting material

2012–2013 admissions summary

	Number of Applicants	Number of New Entrants
Resident	294	49
Nonresident	454	54
Total:	748	103

Expenses for the 2012–2013 Academic Year

Tuition and fees

Resident	$47,055.00
Nonresident	$47,055.00

University of Wisconsin

Office of Academic Affairs
School of Veterinary Medicine
2015 Linden Drive
University of Wisconsin-Madison
Madison WI 53706-1102
Telephone: (608) 263-2525
www.vetmed.wisc.edu/oaa

The University of Wisconsin is located in Madison, the state capital, which has a population of about 230,000. Consistently ranked among the nation's "most livable" cities, its hilly terrain, scattered parks, and woodlands saturate the urban setting with a friendly neighborhood atmosphere. Centered on a narrow isthmus among 4 scenic lakes, the city is a recreational paradise. The university sprawls over 900 acres along Lake Mendota and its student population is nearly 45,000. It has rated among the top 10 universities academically since 1910 and is third in the country in volume of research activity.

The School of Veterinary Medicine facility has a modern veterinary medical teaching hospital, modern equipment, and high-quality lab space for teaching and research. The curriculum provides a broad education in veterinary medicine with learning experiences in food animal medicine and other specialty areas. The school pioneered a unique senior rotation in ambulatory service for fourth-year students where they experience the life and work of a veterinarian specializing in large-animal medicine by working in one of 22 practices near Madison. The school has an outstanding research program and many faculty members have joint appointments with the College of Agriculture, the School of Medicine and Public Health, the Regional Primate Center, the McArdle Cancer Research Institute, the National Wildlife Health Laboratory, and the North Central Dairy Forage Center. These outside links provide research and job opportunities for students.

Application Information

To apply for admission, all applicants must complete three (3) online applications: 1) VMCAS, due October 2, 2013 (1 p.m., EDT); 2) Wisconsin's Required Data Form, due October 1, 2013 (1 p.m., EDT) and located at our website: http://www.vetmed.wisc.edu/home; and 3) Wisconsin's Supplemental Application. All applicants will be notified by e-mail in November 2013 to complete our electronic supplemental application and to announce its deadline. Interviews are not required.

For specific application information (availability, deadlines, fees, and VM-CAS participation), please refer to the contact information listed above.

Residency implications: between 60 and 70 Wisconsin residents will be accepted. Wisconsin has no contractual agreements, but may accept 10–20 non-residents. Applicants who can claim legal residency or domicile in more than one state should contact the school.

Prerequisites for Admission

Applicants must complete a minimum of 60 semester credits of college coursework. The 60 credits include the required 40–43 credits of coursework listed below, plus a minimum of 17 credits of elective coursework left to the student's discretion. The 17 elective credits allow the student to meet personal and academic goals and objectives while preparing for admission to veterinary school.

Course requirements and semester hours

General biology or zoology, introductory animal biology course (with laboratory)	5
General and qualitative chemistry, 2-semester lecture series (with laboratory)	8
Organic chemistry, 1-semester lecture satisfying biochemistry prerequisite	3
Biochemistry (organic chemistry must be prerequisite)	3
English composition or journalism	6

Must include completion of:
- satisfactory score on a college English placement exam, or
- an introductory English composition course,

plus completion of one of the following:
- an English composition or journalism course graded on the basis of writing skills, or
- evidence that writing skills were included in the grading of a specific college-level course

Genetics or animal breeding, must include principles of heredity and preferably molecular mechanisms	3
General physics, 2-semester lecture series	6
Statistics, introductory course	3
Social sciences/humanities, any elective courses in social science or the humanities	6

Required undergraduate GPA: A minimum grade of C (2.0) must be earned in all required courses, including courses completed after application. The mean cumulative GPA for the class of 2016 was 3.67 for residents and 3.78 for non-residents.

AP credit policy: must appear on official college transcripts and be equivalent to the appropriate college-level coursework.

Course completion deadline: all coursework must be completed no later than the spring 2014 term prior to admission to the fall 2014 term. Applicants can have no more than four outstanding required courses at the time of application, with no more than two of those four to be completed during the spring semester. Applicants are encouraged to prepare themselves for the DVM curriculum by taking additional upper-level science courses such as anatomy, physiology, microbiology, or cell/molecular biology.

Standardized examinations: Graduate Record Examination (GRE®), general test, is required. All applicants are required to take or retake the GRE, including the writing assessment. The GRE may be taken no later than October 1, 2013. The admissions committee will use the concordance tables provided by ETS. GRE scores must be received by our office no later than October 25, 2013. The mean score for the class of 2016 for the verbal and quantitative portions combined was 1257 for residents and 1318 for nonresidents.

A test of English as a foreign language (TOEFL, MELAB or IELTS scores may be submitted) is required for applicants for whom English is a second language and have not completed an undergraduate education at an English-speaking college or university. The minimum scores accepted are as follows: internet TOEFL=100, computer TOEFL=250, paper TOEFL=600, MELAB=84, IELTS=7. This must be taken no later than **October 1, 2013**. Please see Web site for additional information.

Additional requirements and considerations
    Veterinary medical experience
    Animal contact and work experience
    Other preparatory experience
    College degrees earned
    Extracurricular activities
    Recommendations/evaluations (3 required)
    Honors/awards
    Diversity of background and experiences
    Personal statement

Summary of Admission Procedure

Timetable
> VMCAS application deadline: Wednesday, October 2, 2013 at 1:00 p.m.
> Eastern Time
> Interviews: none
> Date acceptances mailed: mid-March
> School begins: late August

Deposit (to hold place in class): none required.

Deferments: are considered on an individual basis by the Admissions Committee and may be granted for extenuating circumstances.

Evaluation criteria
There is a 2-part admission procedure. For the fall 2012 application year, the class was selected based upon the following comparative evaluation:

1. *Evaluation of academic record*
   Undergraduate cumulative GPA
   Required course GPA
   Most recent 30 semester credit GPA
   GRE® test scores
2. *Evaluation of personal experience and characteristics*
   Animal and veterinary work experience
   Other preparatory experience (includes extracurricular activities)
   Personal history/academic performance (summary category to include review of academic history, academic achievements, diversity of background, etc.)
   Reference letters

2011–2012 admissions summary

	Number of Applicants	Number of New Entrants
Resident	191	60
Nonresident	770	20
Total:	961	80

Expenses for the 2012–2013 Academic Year

Tuition and fees
Resident	$19,036.24
Nonresident	$25,880.56

Dual-Degree Programs
Combined DVM–graduate degree programs are available.

INTERNATIONAL VETERINARY MEDICAL SCHOOLS

AVMA / COE ACCREDITED

University of Calgary Faculty of Veterinary Medicine Admissions

University of Calgary Faculty of Veterinary Medicine Admissions
TRW 2D03, 3280 Hospital Drive NW
Calgary, AB T2N 4Z6
Telephone: 403.220.8699
Facsimile: 403.210.8121
Email: vet.admissions@ucalgary.ca
Application Deadline: January 10

Doctor of Veterinary Medicine

The University of Calgary Faculty of Veterinary Medicine (UCVM) offers a four-year professional degree leading to a Doctor of Veterinary Medicine (DVM). Completion of at least two years of post-secondary instruction at a recognized university or at a college providing university-equivalency in coursework is required prior to application to the DVM program.

Admissions

Enrolment in the DVM program at UCVM is currently limited to approximately 32 students who are Alberta residents. The Admissions Committee selects students for the program on the basis of academic and non-academic factors. Students are assessed academically on performance in their last four full-time undergraduate terms and in the required courses. Applicants meeting the academic eligibility requirements are invited for an interview day where non-academic factors are assessed. At interview day, applicants are required to complete an on-site essay and participate in a series of interviews and other activities. Applicants must attend interview day at their own expense. There is no entrance exam or requirement to complete the MCAT or GRE exams.

The admissions process identifies applicants who will flourish in a DVM program that prepares students for all aspects of veterinary medicine. Consistent with the UCVM mandate, preference will be given to applicants who demonstrate an interest in pursuing careers in general veterinary practice that support rural development and sustainability, and careers in the areas of emphasis. There is no specific animal or veterinary-related experience required; however, demonstration and understanding of the veterinary profession and animal industries relevant to the applicant's career interests is expected.

Applicants will be notified of the Admissions Committee's decision in June.

Eligibility

At present, applicants must be Alberta residents, as defined by the following rules.

(a) The Residence of an applicant remains that of his/her parent(s) unless a new Residence has been established in accordance with clause (b);

(b) The Residence of an applicant shall be considered to be Alberta, if the applicant has last resided in Alberta for a period of twelve consecutive months (without including any period during which the applicant was attending a college or university) prior to enrolment on the first day of classes;

(c) A Canadian citizen who is resident outside Canada and intends to re-establish residence in Canada shall be considered a resident of the province or territory of Canada where he/she last resided for a period of twelve consecutive months before leaving Canada; and,

(d) A person who is a permanent resident as defined in the Immigration Act (Canada) shall be considered to be a resident of the province or territory where he or she first landed unless the person is considered to be a resident of another province or territory of Canada pursuant to clause (b).

The Faculty of Veterinary Medicine does not normally accept applications from students who have withdrawn, who have been required to withdraw, or who have been expelled from any school or college of veterinary medicine.

In selecting veterinary medicine students, no consideration shall be given to factors irrelevant to performance such as gender, race, or religion. Nor will the vocation of an applicant's parent, guardian, or spouse be a consideration in the selection process.

Minimum Academic Requirements

Normally, the minimum academic requirements for an applicant to receive consideration for an admissions interview are:

(a) Completion of, or in the final semester of completion of, at least two years of full time post-secondary instruction at a recognized university or at a college providing university-equivalency in coursework. A full academic year is defined as a minimum of 4 courses per semester and 2 complete semesters, September - April (16 half-course equivalents).

(b) Completion of, or in the final semester of completion of, the following ten required courses, with a minimum combined average of 2.7 (B- or its equivalent) and a passing grade in each course. Prerequisite courses may only be repeated once to be considered in the admissions process.

Biology:	Two introductory Biology courses
Genetics:	One introductory Genetics course
Ecology:	One introductory Ecology course
Chemistry:	Two introductory Chemistry courses

Organic Chemistry:	One introductory Organic Chemistry course
Biochemistry:	One introductory Biochemistry course
Mathematics:	One introductory Statistics course
English:	One introductory English course

(c) A minimum average of 3.00 (B, or its equivalent) over the last four full undergraduate terms.

(d) Applicants who present required courses that have been taken greater than 10 years prior to the application date will not normally be considered for admission. Exceptions may be made for applicants who have continued to work or study in a health-sciences related field following completion of an undergraduate degree.

Applicants are advised to monitor the UCVM Website for any exceptions or changes to these requirements.

English Language Proficiency

English language proficiency must be demonstrated for all applicants for whom English is not their first language. English language proficiency can be demonstrated in one of the following ways:

(a) Completion of at least two full years within a degree program offered by an accredited university in a country which the University of Calgary recognizes as English language proficiency exempt.

(b) A minimum score of 92 on the internet based TOEFL (Test of English as a Foreign Language) and a minimum score of 50 on the Test of Spoken English (TSE); or a minimum score of 237 on the computer based TOEFL and a minimum score of 50 on the TSE; or a minimum score of 580 on the paper based TOEFL and a minimum score of 50 on the TSE.

Applications

Application forms for the Faculty of Veterinary Medicine are available on the website (vet.ucalgary.ca/dvmprogram). Applications will be considered from those students meeting the residency, English and academic admission requirements. Applications are to be submitted to the UCVM Office of Admissions by January 10th. Two sets of official transcripts are required, one sent in by the first week of February and the second should be sent as soon as final marks are available in the spring and no later than the first week of June. Transcripts should be sent directly to the UCVM Admissions Office. Please refer to the website for the exact deadlines.

Completed application forms include the following: complete personal information; a signed statement verifying Alberta residency status and verifying completion of the academic requirements; three letters of reference (required by January 10th with the application); post-secondary transcripts submitted by the appropriate academic institution; a statement of work experience; and a statement of major extra-curricular activities.

Registration

All successful applicants are required to forward $200.00 deposit within 15 working days of notification of admission. Failure to do so may result in the position being assigned to another applicant. Such deposits will be applied to the first year's fees. An applicant who accepts a position but later rescinds his or her acceptance will forfeit the entire $200.00 deposit.

Successful applicants are required to have or receive immunization for tetanus and rabies following admission.

Accuracy of Registration

The DVM program will register successful applicants and ongoing students into all required yearly courses. Payment of fees is the student's responsibility through the Online Student Centre via My UofC web portal. For more information refer to the "Payment of Fees or Notification of Financial Assistance" in the Registration section of this Calendar.

Deferrals

Students wishing to apply for deferral should make this request in a letter to the UCVM Admissions Office within 15 days of the date at the top of their acceptance letter. Deferrals will be considered for academic and/or non-academic reasons. Deferral requests for attending other veterinary schools will not be accepted. It is at the sole discretion of the Dean to grant or deny a deferral.

University College Dublin
Veterinary Medicine Degree Programme

VMCAS Veterinary Medicine Applications
UCD Admissions Office
Tierney Building
University College Dublin
Belfield, Dublin 4
Ireland
Tel: 00 353 1 716 1555
Email: onlineapps@ucd.ie
http://www.ucd.ie/vetmed/

University College Dublin (UCD) traces its origins to the Catholic University of Ireland founded in 1854 by Cardinal John Henry Newman, author of the celebrated "The Idea of a University." Since then, the University has played a central role in Ireland's advancement as a dynamic and highly successful European state and has established a long and distinguished tradition of service to scholarship and the community.

UCD is the sole provider of a veterinary medicine degree programme on the island of Ireland, and enjoys a long and proud tradition in the provision of veterinary education. Students of the veterinary medicine programme benefit from the outstanding facilities of the purpose-designed UCD Veterinary Sciences Centre and UCD Veterinary Hospital on the main university campus at Belfield, Dublin (commissioned in 2002). Located on a 132 Ha site 5km south of Dublin's City Centre, UCD is Ireland's largest university with over 23,000 students. This is complemented by Lyons Estate Farm where students have practical classes at all stages of the curriculum. The veterinary facilities are state-of-the-art. As part of the UCD College of Agriculture, Food Science & Veterinary Medicine we provide the ideal environment for students and staff to work together to push back the frontiers of knowledge in veterinary research, thus advancing animal health, animal welfare, and human health.

Programme/Syllabus

Our veterinary programme is accredited by the Veterinary Council of Ireland, the American Veterinary Medical Association, and the European Association of Establishments in Veterinary Education. Our programme is designed to educate you to the best international standards in veterinary medicine and to prepare you for entry to any branch of the veterinary profession. Veterinary medicine is concerned with the promotion of the health and welfare of animals of special importance to society. This involves the care of healthy and sick animals, the prevention, recognition, control and treatment of their diseases and the welfare and productivity of livestock. Veterinarians also safeguard human health through prevention and control of diseases transmitted from animals to man, through ensuring the safety of foods of animal origin, and through advancing the science and art of comparative medicine.

Veterinary graduates may work in private practice (companion animals, food animals, horses, exotics, or a mixture of these), in government service (animal health, food safety, public health), in research or in industry.

US applicants through VMCAS are eligible to apply to enter this programme provided they have the prerequisites as outlined below. Further curricular details are published on our web site, www.ucd.ie/vetmed.

The Programme is organised into four stages. During Stage 2 students will take combined modules with students on the Veterinary Medicine programme aimed at school-leavers. In Semesters 1 and 2 of the programme students will build on their knowledge of the basic biological sciences by taking modules designed to demonstrate how this knowledge is applied in the practice of veterinary medicine, and gain a firm grounding in animal welfare, behaviour and handling. A key objective will be to ensure that students have the required knowledge, skills and competences to progress to Stage 2. As the programme progresses students will learn clinical skills and study each of the clinical sciences using a "body systems" approach. Beginning in stage 1 students are required to complete a minimum of 34 weeks of practical extra-mural experience to be completed by stage 4 according to the specifications/regulations for Extra Mural Studies (EMS). The final year of the programme consists of clinical rotations in UCD's veterinary hospital where students have the opportunity to work alongside experienced and specialist staff clinicians, and participate in patient care and client communication. Each student has a personalized timetable ensuring that they participate in rotations in Large and Small Animal Surgeries, Diagnostic Imaging, Anesthesiology, Small and Large Animal Medicine, Emergency Medicine, Clinical Reproduction, Herd Health, Population Medicine, Diagnostic Pathology and Clinical Pathology. Assessments at the end of this clinical year are through Objective Structured Clinical Examinations (OSCEs) and Clinical Proficiency Examinations (CPEs). Throughout the programme students are required to participate in extra-mural studies. In the early years, this consists of gaining experience in the handling and management of farm and companion animals, and in later years, of working with veterinarians in practice (clinical extra-mural experience).

Application Information

For specific application information (availability, fees and VMCAS participation), please refer to the contact information listed above. For further information on entry to the Republic of Ireland, please refer to www.educationireland. ie. Students must also be able to ensure adequate financial support for the duration of their programme.

Prerequisites for Admission

Course requirements

4-Year Graduate Entry Programme

Candidates who have studied and will complete a degree in an appropriate biological science may be considered for the 4- year Graduate programme in Veterinary Medicine with the award of MVB.

Required undergraduate GPA: 3.2 (on 4.0-point scale)

Course completion deadline: all required courses should be completed prior to August of the year of admission.

5-Year Undergraduate Programme MVB: Those candidates with a nonscience degree will be considered for first year entry to the 5-year MVB programme, provided they have gained high grades in the science subjects, including chemistry and biology.

Standardized examinations: none required. GRE® results will be considered if submitted.

Additional requirements and considerations
Applicants are also expected to have gained relevant work experience of handling animals. This should, where possible, include not only seeing veterinary practice, but also spending time on livestock farms and other animal establishments.

Summary of Admission Procedure

Timetable
> VMCAS application deadline: Wednesday, October 2, 2013 at 1:00 p.m.
> Eastern Time
> Date offers mailed: December/January
> Term begins: early September

Deposit (to hold place in class): €2,000 euros, required by early March

Deferments: Not applicable

Evaluation criteria

Academic performance

References/evaluations (minimum 2 required-one from academic science source and one from a veterinary surgeon)

1 page personal statement

Animal & Veterinary Experience

2011-2012 admissions summary (for entry in 2012)

	Number of Applicants	Number of New Entrants
In-province	891	96
International	190	24
Total	1,081	120

Expenses for the 2013-2014*

Annual tuition and fees

EU Graduate	19,500 euros
Non EU Graduate	33,500 euros

Admission Process:

US and Canadian residents must apply to UCD through VMCAS and a supplemental application form which is available at www.ucd.ie/vetmed

Completed applications are reviewed by our admissions team. No interviews will take place. Successful applicants will receive their offers in December/January. Classes begin in early September with compulsory orientation taking place prior to the start of classes.

Entrance Requirements:

Up to 30 places will be available in 2013 for overseas students. We look for a GPA of 3.2 or above.

All additional information required by UCD including the completed online supplemental application and supporting documentation by Friday, 1st November 2013.

* For up-to-date information on fees and all further information regarding admission to the University College Dublin, please visit our web site www.ucd.ie.

University of Edinburgh
Royal (Dick) School of Veterinary Studies

BVM&S Admissions Office
Royal (Dick) School of Veterinary Studies
The University of Edinburgh
Easter Bush Veterinary Centre
Roslin EH25 9RG
Scotland, UK
Tel: +44 (0)131 651 7305
Fax: +44 (0)131 650 6585
Email: geraldine.giannopoulos@ed.ac.uk
http://www.ed.ac.uk/schools-departments/vet

The Royal (Dick) School of Veterinary Studies, established in 1823, was the first veterinary school in Scotland, and the second to be established in the UK. The long-standing involvement of Edinburgh with veterinary education, where tradition is mixed with cutting-edge veterinary teaching, benefits from a closely-knit collegial community of "Dick" vet students. As one of only 14 international vet schools with AVMA accreditation, the veterinary degree course at Edinburgh (BVM&S) provides an excellent foundation for a subsequent career in veterinary practice throughout the world or one of the many related career opportunities, such as biomedical research. The academic and research environment in Edinburgh is internationally recognised for encouraging excellence in a broad base of teaching and learning. The School has a great advantage of being located on one site approximately 7 miles south of the city. The Easter Bush campus incorporates a new, purpose-built £40 million teaching building, small animal, equine and farm animal hospital facilities with both first-opinion and referral services, and the world-renowned Roslin Institute located in a £60 million facility offering opportunities to carry out research supervised by pre-eminent researchers in numerous fields. In addition, Edinburgh has a unique comprehensive exotic and wildlife service.

Clinical training begins at the start of first year in our clinically integrated programme with training in examining normal animals across the common species progressing to abnormal animals in later years. The lecture-free Final Year emphasises small-group practical, clinical experience where students undertake clinical rotations in the School's hospitals and support services giving students practical experience in a wide range of disciplines. The Final Year is longer than the previous years and incorporates an externship and elective periods to allow focus on areas of individual interest. Students also bring together their personal and professional development portfolio which enhances their employability, encourages life-long learning and promotes professionalism.

The city of Edinburgh, the capital of Scotland, is one of Europe's most handsome cities. The beauty of its setting and its architecture, allied with its intellectual traditions, have earned the title of "Athens of the North" for what is still a compact city of some 500,000 people. It is a city of noted buildings, fine gardens, and open spaces, including Holyrood Park—one of the largest city centre natural parks in Europe—and Princes Street Gardens, between the Old and New Towns. The city offers students a rich mix of academic, social and allied facilities—libraries, museums and art galleries, concert halls, theatres and cinemas. The city has easy access to coastline, lochs, mountains and countryside, with ready-made opportunities for open-air sports and recreation.

Further details on the BVM&S degree programme, the School and its facilities can be found by visiting http://www.ed.ac.uk/schools-departments/vet

Application Information

For specific application information (availability, deadlines, fees and VMCAS participation), please refer to the contact information listed above.

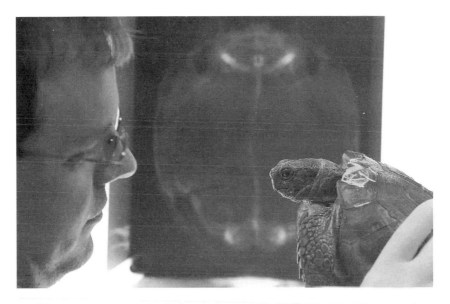

Our Hospital for Small Animals has the largest Exotics department in Europe and our academics are international experts in treating species from around the world. Studying in Edinburgh will allow you to experience the widest variety of cases. Photograph courtesy of School of Veterinary Medicine, The University of Edinburgh

Residency implications: For full details and further information on entry to the UK, please refer to http://www.ukba.homeoffice.gov.uk. Please note that students must be able to ensure adequate financial support for the duration of their course. Candidates are not required to submit a supplemental application.

Prerequisites for Admission

Course requirements

5-Year BVM&S Programme:

Applicants are expected to have completed a minimum of at least 2 years of a preveterinary or science course at college or university. A minimum of one year (2 semesters or 3 terms) in chemistry, and additional courses in biology, physics and/or mathematics are required. All applicants are required to have gained high grades in the science subjects, especially chemistry. U.S. applicants should have an overall minimum grade point average of 3.4 (4-point scale), with greater than 3.0 in science courses which have been completed.

Those candidates with a nonscience degree would be considered for first-year entry to the 5-year BVM&S course, provided they have gained high grades in the science subjects, including chemistry and biology.

4-Year Graduate Entry Programme:

Candidates who have studied and will complete a degree in an appropriate biological science may be considered for the 4-year BVM&S programme (Graduate Entry Programme).

Required undergraduate GPA: 3.4 with greater than 3.0 in science courses (on 4.0-point scale)

Course completion deadline: all required courses should be completed prior to August of the year of admission.

Standardized examinations: Graduate Record Examination (GRE®) general test is required. The scores must be received by November 1 for 2014 entry. Applicants should ensure they take the GRE early enough for scores to be received by the deadline.

Additional requirements and considerations
Applicants are also expected to have gained relevant practical work experience with animals. This should, where possible, include not only seeing veterinary practice, but also spending time on livestock farms and other animal establishments (paid or unpaid experience acceptable).

Summary of Admission Procedure

Timetable
> VMCAS application deadline: Wednesday, October 2, 2013 at 1:00 p.m. Eastern Time
> Receptions: early–mid-February (held in the U.S.)
> Date acceptances mailed: early April at the latest
> School begins: mid-September or early August (for GEP entrants)

Deposit (to hold place in class): £1,500, required by early May

Deferments: Not applicable

Evaluation criteria
> Academic performance
> GRE® scores
> Animal/veterinary experience
> Personal statement
> Motivation
> References/Evaluations (minimum 2 required—one from academic science source and one from a veterinary surgeon)

2011-2012 admissions summary (for entry in 2012)*

	Number of Applicants	Number of New Entrants
In-province	904	72
International	584	101
Total	1,488	173

Expenses for the 2012–2013 Academic Year*

Tuition and fees
Resident	residents of the UK, who do not hold a first degree, are primarily government-funded
International	£27,900 (fixed for duration of course)

* For up-to-date information on fees and all further information regarding admission to the School, please visit our website www.ed.ac.uk/schools-departments/vet

* further information on funding including estimated living costs for international students is available here: http://www.ed.ac.uk/studying/international/finance

University of Glasgow

Mrs. Joyce Wason
Director of Admissions & Student Services Manager
College of Medicine, Veterinary and Life Sciences
School of Veterinary Medicine
Bearsden Road
Bearsden Glasgow G61 1QH
Tel: (+44) 141 330 5705
Fax: (+44) 141 942 7215
Email: vet-sch-admissions@glasgow.ac.uk

As one of the world's top 100 universities, the University of Glasgow combines tradition with academic excellence.

The school is one of only five veterinary schools in Europe to be accredited to British, European and American standards.

Building on more than 140 years of expertise, the School of Veterinary Medicine is at one and the same time a hospital, a research institute and a top-rated teaching establishment, training the next generation of veterinary practitioners and scientists.

It is in a unique position as the only Veterinary School in the UK where all the academic departments are located together. The single site houses pre-clinical and clinical departments, a small animal hospital and the Weipers Centre for Equine Welfare. Cochno Farm & Research Centre, an additional teaching facility, lies just five miles away.

The school has always taken great pride in its innovative teaching programmes and was the first in the UK to establish a totally clinical final year that helps to prepare students thoroughly for the world of work. Teaching is rated as 'excellent' by the latest independent Quality Assessment of Teaching. The school also achieved the highest results among all UK AVMA accredited schools for student satisfaction in the National Student Survey.

2009 saw the completion of a new state of the art £15m Small Animal Hospital and a new £2.5m production animal facility. The current hospital treats over 9,000 cases each year and the number is growing steadily. It provides a referral service to veterinary general practitioners and its staff includes clinicians for all specialities.

The city of Glasgow has a population of around 74,000 and is Scotland's largest city. One of Europe's liveliest places with a varied and colorful cultural and social life, it can cater to every taste. Situated on the River Clyde, Glasgow has excellent road and rail links to the rest of the UK and air services to a wide range of destinations, both home and overseas.

Wherever you come from, you can be sure of building friendships that last a lifetime at Glasgow. According to travel guide Lonely Planet, Glasgow is one of the world's top ten cities.

Application Information

For specific application information (availability, deadlines, fees, and VMCAS participation), please refer to the contact information listed above.

Residency implications: Due to recent changes in immigration legislation, students from the U.S. (who are planning to come to the UK for more than 6 months) are now required to obtain an entry clearance certificate prior to entering the UK. For further information on entry to the UK, please refer to http://www.ukvisas.gov.uk. Students must also be able to ensure adequate financial support for the duration of their course.

Prerequisites for Admission to the Programme

Course requirements
Applicants are expected to have completed at least 2 years pre-veterinary or science courses at College or University, with a minimum of one year in Chemistry (including organic chemistry and organic chemistry lab). We would expect high grades in all science subjects. US applicant should have a minimum 3.4 GPA (4 point scale), and to have achieved at 3.0 in Science.

Required undergraduate GPA: 3.40.

AP credit policy: not applicable.

Course completion deadline: required courses should be completed prior to admission in the fall.

Standardized examinations: none required. GRE® results will be considered if submitted.

Additional requirements and considerations
> Animal/veterinary work experience sufficient to indicate motivation, interest, and understanding of the veterinary profession
> Evaluations: minimum 2, one each from an academic science source and a veterinary surgeon.
> There is no supplemental application for the University of Glasgow.

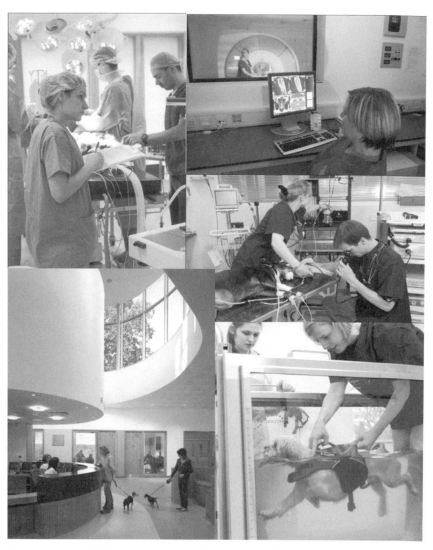

The University of Glasgow offers state-of-the art animal care facilities and first class teaching and research opportunities.

Summary of Admission Procedure

Timetable
>VMCAS application deadline: Wednesday, October 2, 2013 at 1:00 p.m.
>   Eastern Time
>Date interviews held: January/February–(In the US both East and
>   West Coast)
>Date acceptances mailed: April
>School begins: late September

Deposit (to hold place in class): £1,000

Deferments: in certain circumstances.

Evaluation criteria
>Academic performance
>Animal/veterinary experience
>References
>Essay
>Interview

2011–2012 admissions summary

	Number of Applicants	Number of New Entrants
In-province	1,100	72
International	350	55
Total:	1,450	127

Expenses for entry in 2014

Tuition and fees

Resident	Residents of Scotland and EU are Government funded. Students out with these areas are required to pay a top up fee of £9000 per annum
International	£25,000

For further information, contact the Undergraduate School Admissions Office (vet-sch-admissions@glasgow.ac.uk)

University of Guelph

Admissions, Office of Registrarial Services
University Centre, Level 3
University of Guelph
Guelph Ontario N1G 2W1
Canada
Telephone: (519) 824-4120, ext. 56060
www.ovc.uoguelph.ca

Founded in 1862, the Ontario Veterinary College is located in Guelph, Ontario; about 97 miles north of Buffalo. Guelph has a similar climate to Detroit and Chicago. Surrounded by gently rolling farmland and known for its safety, friendly people, warm summers and brisk winters, this city of 120,000 is typical of the northeast.

The university has an enrolment of over 18,000 undergraduate students of which 462 are in the Doctor of Veterinary Medicine (DVM) program. There are also approximately 200 graduate students, 100 faculty and 200 staff members at the veterinary college, which offers degree programs leading to a DVM, MPH, MSc, PhD, Doctor of Veterinary Science (DVSc) and a Graduate Diploma. The college has four departments: Population Medicine, Clinical Studies, Biomedical Sciences; and Pathobiology with 10 million $C in research funding from various government and private sector sources. The site features a full-service teaching hospital with both a large animal and a small animal clinic. There are also large, modern research stations for separately housing sheep, swine, and dairy and beef cattle, and a Centre for Public Health and Zoonoses. In 2010 we opened our new Hill's Pet Nutrition Primary Healthcare Centre, a unique educational centre ensuring OVC will continue to be an international leader in learning, teaching and research in companion animal primary health care and service delivery.

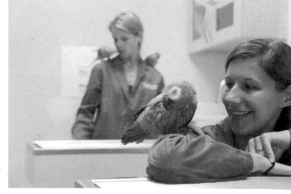

Two third year veterinary medicine students learning avian behaviour at the Ontario Veterinary College.

Application Information

For specific application information (availability, deadlines, fees, and VMCAS participation), please refer to the contact information listed above.

Residency implications: International applicants will be considered provided the applicant does not hold Canadian citizenship, dual citizenship, or permanent resident status in Canada. There is a maximum of 15 international positions available per year. There is a maximum of 105 seats available per year for Canadians: 100 undergraduate and 5 graduate.

Prerequisites for Admission

Course requirements and semester hours: Students must first complete a minimum of two full-time years (four full-time semesters) of university including specific university courses. Students initially apply for admission to a science degree program. For the purpose of DVM admission, a full-time semester will include at least 5 one-semester courses equivalent to 15 credit hours. Once the prerequisite courses are completed successfully, students apply for admission to the DVM Program. The subject matter requirements listed below must have been completed before admission to the DVM program will be considered.

Course requirements and semesters

Biological sciences (emphasis on animal biology)	2
Cell biology	1
Genetics	1
Biochemistry	1
Statistics	1
Humanities or social sciences*	2

* Students entering the DVM program should be able to operate across discipline boundaries recognizing the relevance of the humanities and social sciences to their career choice. In selecting these courses from among those acceptable, the prospective veterinary student should consider topics such as ethics, logic, critical thinking, determinants of human behavior, and human social interaction.

Required courses proposed to be completed at an institution other than the University of Guelph should be approved as acceptable prior to course registration. Applicants are required to request approval for courses in writing. Course descriptions must be included with the request. Courses will not be acceptable if they are repeats of previously passed courses, or if they are taken at the same or a lower level in a subject area than previously passed courses in the same subject area. It is expected that the required undergraduate preparation for the DVM program will be completed in a full-time coherent academic program.

Required undergraduate GPA: students with a minimum GPA of 3.00 on a 4.00 scale based on the cumulative average, average of the required courses and the last two semesters in full-time attendance at university may be further considered.

Course completion deadline: required courses must be completed by August 31 of the year prior to application in order to be further considered. For example for fall 2014 entry courses must be completed by August 31, 2013.

Standardized examinations: Non-Canadian applicants submit Graduate Record Examination (GRE) scores. The code for GRE scores is 0892. For Canadian applicants Medical College Admission Test (MCAT) is required. Test scores must be received no later than December 1 of the year prior to application.

Additional requirements and considerations
> Reasons for choosing a career in veterinary medicine
> Quality of preparatory academic program
> Experience and knowledge in matters relating to animals and to the veterinary medical profession
> Experience and achievement in extracurricular affairs and/or community service activities
> Communication skills
> Three confidential referee assessments comprised of an evaluative form and a letter are required for each DVM applicant. The referees have to be qualified to give an unbiased, informed and critical assessment of the applicant. **Two of the three referees that applicants select must be veterinarians** with whom he or she has obtained veterinary and/or animal experience. There is a strong preference for veterinarians from different clinics.

Supplemental form: An Academic Background Form accompanied by course descriptions is required of all applicants. The Form is available here: http://www.ovc.uoguelph.ca/future/dvm/applicants/non-canadian/documents/Prerequisiteform2014app_000.pdf

Summary of Admission Procedure

Timetable
> VMCAS application deadline: Wednesday, October 2, 2013 at 1:00 p.m. Eastern Time
> Document Deadline: December 1, 2013
> Date interviews are held: November–March
> Date acceptances mailed: November–March
> School begins: September

Please note that late applications will be considered if seats remain open. If you are interested in applying directly to OVC after these deadlines, please contact Elizabeth Lowenger <lowenger@uoguelph.ca>.

Deposit (to hold place in class): A non-refundable deposit of $3,000.00 Cdn is due after an offer of acceptance is made to hold a seat in the class.

2012 admissions summary

	Number of Applicants	Number of New Entrants
Residents	300	105
International Residents	136	11
Total:	436	116

Expenses for the 2012–2013 Academic Year

Tuition and fees
Resident	$8609.50 $C
Visa student	$53 554.58 $C

Massey University

International Student Affairs
Undergraduate Office
Massey University Veterinary School
IVABS
Massey University
Private Bag 11-222
Palmerston North 4442
New Zealand
Tel: (+646) 350 5222
Fax (+646) 350 5654
Email: vetschool@massey.ac.nz
http://vet-school.massey.ac.nz/

The Massey University veterinary program was the first veterinary program to gain AVMA accreditation in Australasia.

The Massey University Veterinary School accepts up to 24 international students annually with a total class size of approximately 100. The first class of Massey veterinarians graduated in 1967, and since then more than 2,500 veterinarians have graduated and are working around the world.

The Massey University veterinary program has an international reputation for providing an excellent veterinary education with a strong science background, a broad knowledge of companion, equine, and production animal health, and a focus on independent thinking and problem-solving skills. The curriculum incorporates practical aspects throughout all years of the degree beginning with animal handling and behaviour in the first post-selection semester through to the final year of the program, which is almost entirely clinically based.

Years 1 and 2 of the program focus primarily on instruction in the core medical sciences tailored for veterinary students to learn normal form and function. In year 3 and 4 classes help the student recognise abnormality and focus on the medicine, surgery, health management, diagnostics and treatment of companion and agricultural animal species. The fifth year is a semi-tracked clinically based year. Each student will choose a track from the following options: small animal, production animal, equine or mixed animal, or other areas as approved (i.e. wildlife, research). All tracks share a core of 18 weeks of rotations covering multiple species, then depending on the track a further 7-9 weeks will be prescribed. The student will then have 7-9 weeks where they can choose to do externships (within New Zealand or overseas), or further clinics at Massey University. The semi-tracked, individualised final year curriculum allows students to further explore their area of interest while ensuring wide coverage of the main veterinary species.

The veterinary facilities are of a high international standard with numerous other university-run animal units (dairy, beef, sheep and deer farms, equine blood typing unit, feline unit, large animal teaching unit, etc.) on or adjacent to the Palmerston North campus. The veterinary teaching hospital sees first-opinion cases as well as referral cases to provide a balanced clinical experience for the students. The Massey University veterinary school staff are collegial, motivated, highly qualified individuals, many of whom are board certified specialists in their discipline.

The vet school is located in Palmerston North, a student-friendly town of 75,000 in the lower central north island of New Zealand. Nicknamed "student city," Palmerston North offers free bus service and bikes to Massey students and is home to numerous cafés, restaurants, bars, theatres, and outdoor recreational activities. Palmerston North is a one-hour flight from Auckland, is conveniently close to west coast beaches, and is just under a two-hour drive to the Hawke's Bay wine region, skiing and snowboarding at Mt Ruapehu and the country's capital city, Wellington. Renowned for an excellent lifestyle, New Zealand is a great place to study abroad for your AVMA accredited veterinary degree.

Application Information

Specific information (availability, deadlines, fees, and VMCAS participation, the supplemental application and direct application) can be found on the Massey University veterinary school website listed in the contact details above.

US and Canadian residents may apply to Massey University by either:
1. VMCAS **and** a supplemental Massey University application or
2. Direct application to Massey University.

All other non-New Zealand residents are to apply directly to Massey University

Residency implications: All non-New Zealand resident students require a student visa, which is easily obtained following an offer of admission into the program. Students must be able to ensure financial support for the duration of their course.

Prerequisites for Admissions

Course requirements

Group 1—Competitive Selection into Vet School via Semester 1 (10-14 places available)

Group 1 applicants come to Massey University to complete a semester (beginning in late February of each year) of full-time science study (4 classes) at Massey University in order to develop a GPA for selection. Credit will be given where similar classes to the four prerequisite classes have already been completed, and alternate science classes will be chosen by the student.

Group 2—Competitive Selection directly into BVSc Semester 2 (10-14 places available)

Applicants are required to have completed at least two full years of full-time, largely science based university education. Applicants need to have passed classes equivalent to the 4 standard Massey University veterinary prerequisite classes:

Massey University Class	Usual classes needed for credit
Chemistry and Living Systems	General chemistry + Organic chemistry
Physics for Life Sciences	1 year of physics
Biology of Cells	Cell (molecular) biology +/– First year biology series
Biology of Animals	Animal biology / vertebrate zoology

Each of the above classes should include laboratories.

Required undergraduate GPA: a minimum science GPA of 3.00 is required to be eligible for selection into the veterinary degree.

Course completion deadline:
> Group 2: all required courses should be completed by the end of the fall semester in the year prior to matriculation (i.e. Fall 2013 for matriculation in 2014).
> Group 1: not applicable; courses completed in New Zealand.

Standardized examinations: Graduate Record Examination (GRE®), general test, is required for Group 2 applicants only. Test scores should be no older than 5 years immediately preceding the application deadline. Scores must be received by the supplemental application deadline (see below).

The STAT-F test is required for Group 1 applicants only. The test will be offered at Massey University in the semester 1 examination period (June). In the uncommon situation that a student sat the STAT-F test elsewhere the deadline for submission of scores would be June 15.

Additional requirements and considerations: All VMCAS applicants must complete the supplemental application for Massey University. Your application will not be processed until we have received your supplemental application. The supplemental application and instructions on completing the application can be found at http://www.massey.ac.nz/massey/learning/departments/institute-veterinary-animal-biomedical-sciences/vetschool/apply/applying-vmcas.cfm

A letter signed by a veterinarian on his/her clinic letterhead verifying you have completed a minimum of 10 days (80 hours) work experience at their clinic.

Letters of recommendation are not required. A bachelor's degree is not a prerequisite requirement for admission into the veterinary degree.

Summary of Admission Procedure

Timetable
  Group 1 (semester 1)
    Application deadline: November 1
    Date letters of admission to semester 1 sent: once completed
      application received and processed.
    School begins: late February (semester 1)
    Date acceptances into the veterinary degree program mailed: early July
    Date veterinary degree program begins: mid-July (semester 2)
  Group 2
    VMCAS application deadline: Wednesday, October 2, 2013 at 1:00 p.m.
      Eastern Time (VMCAS application completed online).
      Supplemental application with all supplementary documents to be
      received by November 1.)
    Direct applicants: November 1 (including all supplementary
      documents)
    Date acceptances mailed: from late December
    School begins: mid-July (semester 2) 2014

Deposit (to hold Group 2 position): $NZ 1,500.00

Deferments: offers of a place in semester 2 of the program are for a single year only. Deferments are not permitted. Deferments of offers of a place in semester 1 of the program (Group 1 applicants) are permitted.

Evaluation criteria
  Group 1
    Weighted GPA   80%
      (Minimum of a B average across all 4 first semester
      classes needed to be eligible for selection).
    Special Tertiary Admissions Test (STAT)   20%
      This is the Australian equivalent to the GRE®
      and is held at Massey University in the June
      examination period at the end of the first
      semester.

Group 2
  Science GPA   50%
  GRE® General Test   50%

2012 admissions summary

	Number of Applicants	Number of New Entrants
Residents	300	77
International		
Group 1	61	20
Group 2	<u>118</u>	<u>4</u>
Total:	479	101

Expenses for the 2013 Academic Year

Tuition
  Resident   residents of New Zealand are government subsidized
  International   Semester 1 $NZ 12,700
                      Semesters 2–9 $NZ 26,250 ($NZ 52,500
                                          per year)

Please note - the above tuition fees are in NZ dollars. The actual cost in your currency will depend on the exchange rate at the time of paying tuition fees. The NZD is traditionally substantially lower than USD and CAD.

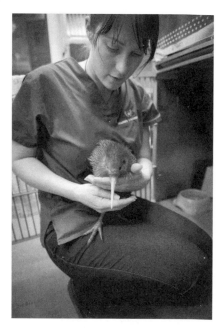

Veterinary student tending to a kiwi at Wildbase, the wildlife hospital of New Zealand based at the Massey University Veterinary School.

The University of Melbourne

Admissions Office
The Faculty of Veterinary Science
The University of Melbourne
Corner Park Drive and Flemington Road
Parkville
3010
Melbourne
Victoria
Australia
Tel: + (613) 8344 7357
Fax: + (613) 8344 7374
www.vet.unimelb.edu.au

The University of Melbourne has a 150 year history of leadership in research, innovation, teaching and learning. As a University of Melbourne student, you will become part of a dynamic collegial environment with a distinctive research edge. Throughout its history the University of Melbourne has educated some of the world's most eminent scientists and researchers and this tradition continues today.

The Faculty of Veterinary Science was the very first veterinary school established in Australia, and celebrated its centenary in 2009. It is concentrated on two sites: the city-centre University campus in Parkville and the Werribee campus, where students study in a state-of-the-art teaching hospital designed to support top-class veterinary education in the 21st century. Facilities include ten consulting rooms, modern diagnostic capabilities including endoscopy, CT, MRI, image intensification, scintigraphy, on-site diagnostic pathology laboratories and a 24-hour small animal emergency and critical care unit.

The veterinary program is made up of industry-linked learning, practical components and internship opportunities. Students gain experience in animal handling, care and management and undertake professional work experience between semesters and academic years, as well as having hands-on experience throughout the course. The school has strong programs in small animal medicine, equine, dairy cattle, sheep and beef cattle medicine.

The degree is accredited by the American Veterinary Medical Association (AVMA), by the Royal College of Veterinary Surgeons (UK), and by the Australasian Veterinary Boards Council Inc. These accreditations reflect the high quality and international standing of the course and permits graduates of the course to work as veterinarians in a wide range of countries including North America.

Our success has been achieved by insisting on international excellence. Talented people from all over the world come to visit, study and work at the University of Melbourne. At last count, the University's student community of 44,000 included more than 9,800 international students from over 100 countries.

We invite you to join our tradition and discover why staff and students of the highest calibre are attracted to study at the Faculty of Veterinary Science at the University of Melbourne.

Course duration, entry routes and student numbers

From 2011 the University of Melbourne offers studies in veterinary education through our newly created professional entry graduate degree; the Doctor of Veterinary Medicine. The new four-year degree will offer veterinary students the best possible preparation for twenty-first century careers in a rapidly changing and increasingly global workforce. As a result of this change, students can enter the veterinary science program by one of two pathways:

1. Students can apply for entry into the three-year Bachelor of Science degree at the University of Melbourne. After completing prerequisite first and second year subjects, students will apply for selection to the Veterinary Bioscience specialisation of the Animal Health and Disease major that will be offered in the third year of the Bachelor of Science. Students who successfully complete all studies in the Veterinary Bioscience specialisation and who successfully complete the Bachelor of Science overall will have guaranteed entry to the DVM program with 100 points' credit (one year of DVM study).

2. Students can also complete a science degree at the University of Melbourne or another institution, and then apply for entry to the DVM at the University of Melbourne. Students will need to have studied at least one semester in each of general or cellular biology and biochemistry within their science degree. Students who follow this pathway will enter the four-year graduate-entry DVM program.

Number of international students that we accept

We currently accept up to 50 international students from across the globe.

Prerequisites for Admission

1. Entrance to the DVM via the Melbourne Bachelor of Science: North American students should refer to the University's international prospectus for up to date details about entrance requirements for the Bachelor of Science by visiting http://futurestudents.unimelb.edu.au/.

166

After completing prerequisite first and second year subjects in the Bachelor of Science, students will be eligible to apply for entry to the Veterinary Bioscience specialisation of the Animal Health and Disease major in third year. Students who successfully complete all studies in the Veterinary Bioscience specialisation will have guaranteed entry into the DVM, with 100 points' credit (one year of study), leaving three years of study in the DVM.

2. Entrance to the DVM as a graduate: Applicants will require a science degree from the University of Melbourne or another institution. Examples of appropriate degrees include Bachelor's degrees with majors in: Agriculture, Animal Science, Biochemistry, Biomedicine, Physiology or Zoology. Prerequisites for entry as a graduate are at least one semester of study in each of general or cellular biology and biochemistry as part of a science degree.

3. There is no standardised test required.

Application Information

International applications will be accepted throughout the year. Applications close on 20 December, commencing enrolment into the following year, however, this is subject to places still being available. Applicants are advised to apply as soon as possible to avoid disappointment. Applications will be considered as soon as they are received. We recognise the amount of time required by successful applicants to make arrangements for international travel and study and we try to give them as much advance notice as possible.

Students apply via the International Admissions Office at the University of Melbourne. They can choose to apply online, download an application form, apply through one of our overseas representatives or request an undergraduate application form to be posted to them. Visit http://futurestudents.unimelb.edu.au/info/international.

Tuition fees: For information about tuition fees please visit http://future students.unimelb.edu.au/admissions/fees to access the University's fee tables for international students.

Application fee: AUD$100.

Visas: All non-Australian students require a student visa, which is easily obtained following an offer of admission into our program. More information can be viewed on the web site: http://services.unimelb.edu.au/international/visas/apply.

Deferments: Please note that successful applicants may not defer commencement of the DVM. Students can reapply for a start year intake when they are able to commence studies, and the application fee will be waived for international students.

For more specific information including fee information please refer to the contact information listed above.

National Autonomous University of Mexico (UNAM) College of Veterinary Medicine

Office of Undergraduate Studies (División de Estudios Profesionales)
College of Veterinary Medicine (FMVZ)
Av. Universidad 3000
Circuito Interior
Delegación Coyoacán
México D.F. 04510
Telephone: 56 22 58 80
Webpage: www.fmvz.unam.mx, http://escolar.fmvz.unam.mx

Email: fmvyz@galois.dgae.unam.mx The College of Veterinary Medicine is located in the south of the main UNAM campus of Mexico City's metropolitan area.

Application Information

Undergraduate admission of new students to the National Autonomous University of Mexico (UNAM) is done through the General Administration Scholar Affairs Direction (DGAE).

The applicants to the College of Veterinary Medicine, students are evaluated in terms of their general academic background, with emphasis on Biology, Chemistry, Physics and Mathematics.

There are two annual applications dates: January and April. Information for specific applications dates can be reviewed at www.escolar.unam.mx (the semester starts in August).

Application forms can be found at the same website. The number of available positions is 450, without distinction for Mexican or foreign applicants.

Residency implications: There are no resident implications. All the students have to take the admission test. Recommendation letters are not needed.

Prerequisites for Admission

Applicants must have at least a high school average grade of 70%.

Minimum of semesters needed in: mathematics, physics, chemistry, and biology

CURSES (Semesters)
Mathematics (4 semesters)
Physics (4 semesters)
Inorganic and organic chemistry (4 semesters)
Principles of biology and general biology (4 semesters)
Social sciences / humanities (6 semesters)

Electives (2 semesters): selected topics on biology, statistics, morphophysiology or physicochemistry

For students from foreign high schools, beside the admission test, they have to submit all necessary official documents to "Dirección General de Incorporación y Revalidación de Estudios (DGIRE) UNAM". Submission instructions can be found at http://www.dgire.unam.mx/contenido/revalidacion/revalbachc.html.

Foreign students whose primary language is not Spanish will have to do a proficiency Spanish language test.

Required undergraduate GPA: It is not necessary

AP credit policy: Is not part of the admission requirements

Course completion deadline: It is based on the application dates, in January and June.

Standardized Examinations: They are not used

Additional requirements and considerations: Foreign students must have a good command of the Spanish language

Summary of Admission Procedure

Timetable
    The next application dates can be checked at www.escolar.unam.mx

Deposit: It is not necessary

Deferments: Considered on an individual basis, and ordinarily granted for personal reasons, illness, lack of economic resources or other situations beyond the control of the students.

Evaluation criteria: Grade of 80% or above in the admission exam.

2012–2013 admissions summary

Number of Applicants	Number of New Entrants
2,742	99 (3.6%)

Expenses for the 2012–2013 Academic Year (subject to change)

Tuition and fees
    $2,000 USD per year

Dual-Degree Program
Does not apply

Leadership Program
Does not apply

Université de Montréal

Service de l'admission et du recrutement
Université de Montréal
C.P. 6205
Succursale Centre-Ville
Montréal Québec H3C 3T5
Canada
Telephone: (514) 343-7076
Email: saefmv@medvet.umontreal.ca
www.medvet.umontreal.ca

Application Information

Applications available: December
   On line: 90$
   Paper: 120$

Application deadline: February 1

Residency implications: Canadian citizenship or permanent residency in Canada is required.

A total of 90 students are admitted each year.

Prerequisites for Admission

DEC (Diplôme d'Etudes Collégiales) including the following courses:

Cours/Course requirements

Physics	101, 201, 301–78
Chemistry	101, 201, 202
Biology	301, 401
Mathematics (including calculus)	103, 203

To be considered for admission, one must: a) have completed the above requirements, or b) have completed equivalent studies.

Note: All lectures are given in French. Examinations must be written in French.

The DMV is a 5-year program.

Condition concerning the knowledge of French: To be admissible, the candidate must demonstrate that he/she has acquired the minimal level of proficiency in French as required by the chosen program, as established by the University. To this end, the candidate must either:

- succeed the Épreuve uniforme de langue et littérature française of the Ministry of Education of Quebec or;

- obtain a score of at least 785/990 on the International French exam (Test de français international TFI) http://www.etudes.umontreal.ca/programme/doc_prog/section2.pdf.

Performance Score: This score is obtained by comparing the student's grade in each course with the class average.

Course completion deadline: The applicant must have completed all prerequisites at the time of application.

Additional considerations (in order of importance)
1. Academic record
2. Interview: the interview is designed to verify the transversal competencies.

Summary of Admission Procedure

Timetable
  Application deadline: February 1
  Interviews: beginning of May
  Notification of acceptance: end of May, early June
  Fall semester begins: end of August
Deposit (to hold place in class): 200 $C.

Evaluation criteria	%
Performance score	60
Interview	40

Estimated Expenses for the 2011–2012 Academic Year

Tuition and fees:	72.26 $C	per credit for residents of Quebec (approx. 45 per year)

195.27 $ per credit for Canadian non-residents of Quebec

Murdoch University

Murdoch International
Murdoch University
South Street
Murdoch 6150
Western Australia
Tel: (61-8) 9360 6000
Fax: (61-8) 9360 6491
Email: internat@murdoch.edu.au
http://www.murdoch.edu.au/School-of-Veterinary-and-Biomedical-Sciences/

Western Australia is known for its brilliant blue skies, warm sunny climate and white sandy beaches. It is a land blessed with some of the world's most precious natural phenomena including the dolphins of Monkey Mia, the 350-million-year-old Bungle Bungle range and the towering karri forests of the South West. Sophisticated yet uncomplicated, the lifestyle for the residents of Perth is relaxed and focuses on the outdoors. There are wineries, beaches, bushland, and unique wildlife within easy reach of the city, and a cosmopolitan mix of cafes, restaurants, pubs and thriving nightlife in the city centre.

Veterinary Science is a five year double degree (Bachelor of Science and Bachelor of Veterinary Medicine and Surgery) designed to impart the knowledge and skills necessary for the diagnosis, treatment and prevention of disease and production problems in pets, farm animals, wildlife and laboratory animals. Veterinary students learn in a true practice atmosphere with the final year of study lecture-free and devoted entirely to clinical exposure, including time spent at Perth Zoo. Murdoch students have access to state-of-the art facilities, all on the one campus, including a 24-hour emergency clinic, large and small animal practices, a well-stocked farm and an equine hospital as well as a production animal ambulatory service.

The curriculum keeps Murdoch at the forefront of veterinary education worldwide. This curriculum allows more time for students to develop areas of special interest through non-core rotations, special topics, externships and extramural experience. A Veterinary Professional Life stream is integrated throughout the course to assist students in their transition to future careers in veterinary science and provides a strong focus for developing professional life skills within the veterinary profession. An Animal Systems stream will allow strengthening and integration of animal production, animal ethics, animal welfare, animal behaviour, biosecurity and veterinary public health throughout the veterinary program.

The veterinary science degree is accredited by the American Veterinary Medical Association (AVMA), the Royal College of Veterinary Surgeons (UK), and the Australian Veterinary Boards Council. Completing your Veterinary Science degree Murdoch saves you years of study, and potentially thousands of dollars; this is because with the correct preparation, the course can be entered into after only one year of tertiary study. Once you have finished your degree at Murdoch, you are eligible to sit your exams with the AVMA just as you would if you completed your studies in North America.

Application Information

For specific information (availability, deadlines, fees, and VMCAS participation), please refer to the contact information listed above.

All non-residents require a student visa, which is easily obtained following an offer of admission into the veterinary course. Applicants whose first language is not English must demonstrate competency in the English language.

Admission Requirements

Students that have completed one or more years of tertiary study are eligible to apply for entry into the five year Veterinary course. Your first year of tertiary study must include units in Chemistry, Cell Function/Biology, and Statistics. Applications are still accepted from school leavers, with high achievers offered a guaranteed place in the veterinary course, provided they study and pass their first year of tertiary education at Murdoch University. It is recommended such students enroll in Animal Science within the School.

Other applicants will be formally selected from those who have successfully completed one year or more of formal tertiary study, including the prerequisite units listed above. Applicants are required to supply with the application form a typed Personal Statement of up to 500 words to which should be attached documents such as curriculum vitae and references, and which should out-line:

- why you wish to become a Veterinarian;
- how you consider your past study and experience to date will assist you to succeed in the veterinary course and as a Veterinarian.

- If you have any fails/late withdrawals in your post-secondary/tertiary study, you should explain the circumstances for your poor performance and why those circumstances will not apply to your Murdoch studies.

- You should aim to demonstrate your motivation and preparation for veterinary science.

Assessment of the application will be based on the academic standard achieved in all previous tertiary study, the personal statement, and evidence of recent veterinary and animal related experience. Depending on whether an applicant has satisfied the prerequisites, an offer will be made directly into the veterinary course. If not, an offer will be made into another course within the School of Veterinary and Biomedical Sciences with an assured progression into the veterinary course after successful completion of that year.

Summary of Admission Procedure

Timetable

> There are four application deadlines each year, which are: March 31, June 30, September 30, and November 30. University first semester teaching begins in mid-February. A few candidates may be eligible to begin in second semester in early August.
> School begins: mid-February.
> Some candidates may be eligible to begin in early August.
>
> VMCAS application deadline: Wednesday, October 2, 2013 at 1:00 p.m. Eastern Time. Please note: If VMCAS application module is not open, students are able to apply directly to Murdoch University. Application form can be found at http://www.murdoch.edu.au/Future-students/International-students/Applying-to-Murdoch/Application-forms/

Deposit to hold a position: $1,000 AUD payable upon acceptance of offer

Expenses for the 2013 Academic Year

Tuition fees:
  Animal Science first year A$27,000* pa
  Veterinary Science A$46,000 pa

Deferments: Considered on merit

*Murdoch University is offering the International Discoverers' Scholarship Scheme in 2013 – please visit Murdoch International website for further information

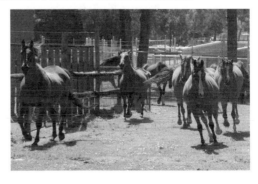

Why look further: Hands on experience right here on our campus.

University of Prince Edward Island

Registrar's Office
Atlantic Veterinary College
University of Prince Edward Island
550 University Avenue
Charlottetown PEI C1A 4P3
Canada
Telephone: (902) 566-0781
Email: registrar@upei.ca
www.upei.ca/registrar/

The Atlantic Veterinary College (AVC), one of the newest colleges of veterinary medicine in North America, opened in 1986 and is fully accredited by the American Veterinary Medical Association, the Canadian Veterinary Medical Association, and the Royal College of Veterinary Surgeons (UK).

Centrally located on Canada's eastern seaboard (650 miles northeast of Boston), the Atlantic Veterinary College makes its home in a beautiful island setting in Charlottetown, Prince Edward Island. With a population of 138,000, which jumps to over a million during the summer tourist season, the community enjoys a small-town lifestyle that boasts the amenities of larger cities, including dining and theatre. Residents also enjoy outdoor activities, such as golfing, cycling, sailing, and cross-country skiing.

The college is a completely integrated teaching, research, and service facility. The four-story complex contains the veterinary teaching hospital, diagnostic services, fish health unit, farm services, postmortem services, animal barns, laboratories, classrooms, computer and audio-visual facilities, offices, cafeteria, and study areas.

Prince Edward Island is a scenic province with a wide variety of dairy, beef, hog, sheep, horse, and fish farms. The combination and variety of animal and fish farms have allowed AVC to develop a special expertise in fish health, aquaculture, and population medicine.

Application Information

For specific application information (availability, deadlines, fees, and VMCAS participation), please refer to the contact information listed above.

Residency implications: Atlantic Veterinary College contracts with New Brunswick (13), Newfoundland (3), Nova Scotia (16), and the home province P.E.I. (10). International students are admitted on a noncontract basis (up to 21).

Prerequisites for Admission

The preveterinary program leading to admission at the Atlantic Veterinary College will normally be completed within the context of a 2-year science program.

Course requirements

Twenty 1-semester courses or equivalent are required. Normally, these courses must be completed while the applicant is enrolled as a full-time student carrying at least 3 courses per semester, at a minimum of 9 semester hours' credit excluding labs. Science courses will normally have a laboratory component and be completed within 6 years of the date of application. Exceptional circumstances will be given consideration; however, it is necessary for all applicants to demonstrate the ability to master difficult subject matter in the context of full-time activity.

Courses must include:

Mathematics	1 course
Statistics	1 course
Biological sciences	2 courses, with labs (emphasis on Animal Biology*)
Microbiology	1 course with lab
Genetics	1 course
Chemistry	3 courses with labs, one being Organic Chemistry
Physics	1 course with lab
English	2 courses, one being English Composition
Humanities and social sciences	3 courses
Electives	5 courses from any discipline

* Examples of animal biology courses include first-year general biology, vertebrate anatomy, vertebrate histology, vertebrate physiology, vertebrate zoology, molecular biology, and cell biology.

Applicants are encouraged to work towards an undergraduate degree. It is recommended that applicants consider including courses in the following topics in their preveterinary curriculum: personal finance, small business management, psychology, sociology, biochemistry, ethics, and logic.

Required undergraduate GPA: no minimum stated (under review as stated above); mean cumulative GPA of most recent entering class is 3.70 on a 4.00 scale.

AP and IB credit policy: a maximum of 6 credits accepted.

Course completion deadline: June 1 of the year of application.

Standardized examinations: Graduate Record Examination (GRE®)

If a student's native language or language of prior education is not English, then the student will be required to pass one of the following: TOEFL, MELAB, IELB, or CanTest.

Additional requirements and considerations
>   Animal/veterinary experience
>   Interview—assessing noncognitive skills
>   Extracurricular activities

Summary of Admission Procedure

Timetable
>   VMCAS application deadline: Wednesday, October 2, 2013 at 1:00 p.m. Eastern Time; November 1 for supplementary application; and January 1 for transfer
>   Date interviews are held: February–March
>   Date acceptances mailed: April
>   School begins: late August; registration, early September

Deposit (to hold place in class): 500.00 $C

Deferments: are considered on a case-by-case basis.

Evaluation criteria
Academic credentials including the GRE are evaluated by the Registrar's Office. Other criteria and activities are evaluated by the admissions committee through an interview process, and the supplementary application.

	% weight
Academic ability	55
Noncognitive ability	35
Veterinary experience	10

2008–2009 admissions summary

	Number of Applicants	Number of New Entrants
In-Province	20	10
Contract*	86	32
International	269	21
Total:	375	63

* For further information, see the listing of contracting states and provinces.

Expenses for the 2012–2013 Academic Year

Tuition and fees
    Resident   *12,308 $C
    Contract student   *12,308 $C
    International student   *54,759 $C (51,500 $US est.)

* For further information, see the listing of contracting states and provinces.

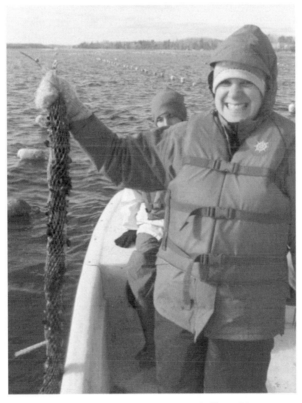

Photo courtesy of Atlantic Veterinary College, University of Prince Edward Island.

University of Queensland

School of Veterinary Science
University of Queensland – Gatton Campus
GATTON, 4343, AUSTRALIA
P: 61 7 5460 1834
F: 61-7 5460 1922
E: vetenquires@uq.edu.au
W: http://www.uq.edu.au/vetschool/

The School

The School of Veterinary Science taught its first class in 1936 and has since educated and trained over 3,000 veterinarians to enter a broad range of careers. The School is located on UQ's Gatton Campus, a 2,600-acre farm some 50 miles west of the capital city of Queensland, Brisbane. Our facilities are excellent, following the $100m construction of new School facilities as part of the School's 2010 relocation to Gatton from Brisbane. The School has full accreditation with the Australasian Veterinary Boards Council, the Royal College of Veterinary Surgeons, and the American Veterinary Medical Association.

The School of Veterinary Science occupies four new buildings that contain companion animal and equine hospitals; veterinary teaching laboratories (dry and wet labs, pathology suite); a four-story office and research tower; and a clinical studies centre that includes a teaching surgery and small animal teaching and research facilities.

The School has four veterinary hospitals and clinics located on three UQ sites. The equine and companion animal hospitals are located centrally on the UQ Gatton Campus. A satellite clinic is located in the rural town of Dayboro 97 km (60 miles) north east of Gatton campus, or about an hour and a half's drive thorough picturesque grazing countryside. Livestock clinical work operates from both the Gatton and Dayboro sites. A third clinic is located on the main St. Lucia campus in Brisbane.

The Veterinary Medical Centre was opened in 2010 and includes 5600m^2 Companion Animal and Equine Hospitals. They feature large consultation rooms, diagnostic imaging services, surgical and medical procedure rooms, tutorial rooms, kennels, stables, and separately located isolation facilities. The Companion Animal Hospital provides GP and specialist services for companion animals and exotic animals including after-hours services. The equine hospital has a predominantly referral caseload and offers 24-hour care.

There are extensive production animal facilities on the Gatton Campus, including an undercover, custom-designed Beef Cattle Teaching Facility, a 200 head feedlot, 400 sow commercial piggery, a dairy with a 250 milking cow capacity, and a poultry facility.

Veterinary students have full access to facilities and services at the Gatton Campus, including six modern lecture theatres with a capacity for 120 students, seminar/tutorial rooms, library, IT facilities, campus-wide wireless Internet, on-campus accommodation, student services, sporting, and social amenities.

The Program

The UQ BVSc degree is a very demanding five-year program. You will develop a comprehensive understanding of the science behind veterinary practice. This knowledge will underpin the technical skills in medicine and surgery that you will need to practise as a veterinarian. UQ graduates must learn all aspects of veterinary science and the skills required to diagnose and treat diseases in the full range of domestic species, as well as native and exotic animals. There is also a requirement to understand public health (including abattoir and biosecurity processes) and preventative medicine.

Admission Requirements

Applicants from outside Australia must apply through UQ International: http://www.uq.edu.au/international/.

Program details, including current costs, can be found at http://www.uq.edu.au/study/program.html?acad_prog=2036#international, or by going to the Courses and Programs link, typing in "Veterinary Science," and selecting International.

Prerequisites

Queensland senior secondary school (or equivalent) English, Chemistry, Mathematics B PLUS either Physics or Biology. International students from non-English speaking countries must have minimum IELTS scores as follows: overall 7; writing 6; speaking 7.

International students must undertake this program on campus at UQ on a full-time basis to be eligible to apply for an Australian student visa. Please contact UQ International.

Closing date

To commence study in semester 1 - November 15 of the previous year for Category 1 and 2 countries; October 15 of the previous year for Category 3 and 4 countries.

This program is eligible for Streamlined Visa Processing.

Please check your country's category with the Department of Immigration and Citizenship: http://www.immi.gov.au/.

Ross University School of Veterinary Medicine

Office of Admissions
Ross University School of Veterinary Medicine
630 US Highway 1
North Brunswick, NJ 08902
Toll-free telephone: 1-855-ROSSVET
Fax: 732-509-4803
Email: Admissions@RossU.edu
www.RossU.edu

Located in St. Kitts, West Indies, Ross University School of Veterinary Medicine (RUSVM) offers an American Veterinary Medical Association (AVMA)-accredited veterinary program focused on educating tomorrow's leaders and discoverers in veterinary medicine. RUSVM is dedicated to providing academic excellence for students as the foundation for becoming sought-after, practice-ready veterinarians for North America and beyond, and has over 2,900 graduates who are successfully practicing veterinary medicine across the US and Canada.

The seven-semester pre-clinical curriculum is enhanced by hands-on clinical experience to help prepare students for the final year of clinical training at one of RUSVM's affiliated veterinary hospitals in the United States. RUSVM's faculty have outstanding credentials in teaching and research and share a passion for educating the veterinarians of tomorrow. RUSVM operates on a three-semester per year calendar.

Each semester is 15 full academic weeks, including final exams. RUSVM graduates are eligible to practice veterinary medicine in all 50 States, Canada and Puerto Rico upon completion of the requisite licensing requirements. RUSVM students who are U.S. citizens/permanent residents and meet the Department of Education qualifying criteria may be eligible for Federal Stafford Loans and Federal Graduate PLUS Loans.

Application Information

For specific application information (availability, deadlines, fees, VMCAS participation, and supplemental application requirements), please refer to the contact information listed above.

Evaluation Criteria:
- Undergraduate cumulative grade point average (GPA)
- GPA in required pre-veterinary course work

- Advanced science courses
- Graduate Record Examination (GRE) scores
- Personal essay
- Letters of recommendation from academic and/or professional references
- Extracurricular activities and accomplishments
- Personal qualities
- Personal interview
- Record of experience working with animals

Prerequisites for Admission

Course Requirements and semester hours:

Biology (General or Zoology) with laboratory	2 semesters or 8 credit hours
Chemistry (General or Inorganic) with laboratory	2 semesters or 8 credit hours
Organic Chemistry with laboratory	1 semester or 4 credit hours
Physics with laboratory	1 semester or 4 credit hours
Biochemistry	1 semester or 3 credit hours
Advanced Biology	3 semesters or 12 credit hours
English*	2 semesters or 6 credit hours
Mathematics	1 semester or 3 credit hours

* Canadian students may satisfy the English requirement using year 13 English or Composition.

Course completion deadline: Required courses must be completed prior to enrollment.

AP credit policy: Must appear on official college transcripts.

Standardized Examinations: Results of the Graduate Record Examination (GRE) are required. Applicants presenting fewer than 60 upper division credits from an English language college or university must provide the official record of the scores for the Test of English as a Foreign Language (TOEFL). The minimum acceptable score is 550 on the paper-based test, or 213 on the computer-based test.

Additional requirements and considerations: It is highly desirable that applicants complete the equivalent of at least six weeks of full-time practical experience, working with large domesticated animals (e.g., cows, horses, sheep, goats, pigs) and small domestic animals (e.g., dogs, cats). It is preferable that all such experience has taken place under the supervision of a practicing veterinarian, but comparable experience may be considered.

Summary of Admission Procedure

Timetable
>Application deadline: None; rolling admissions
>Date interviews are held: Year-round
>Date acceptances mailed: As soon as possible after the interview
>School begins: Three start dates per year: September, January and May

Application fee: $100

Deposit (to hold place in class): $1,000

Deferments: Considered

Tuition for the 2012-2013 Academic Year (subject to change)
>Nonresident $16,800/per semester

For comprehensive consumer information visit www.RossU.edu/vet-student-consumer-info.

Dual-Degree Program

RUSVM has dual degree agreements with several undergraduate institutions. Under this program, any undergraduate junior who meets the set standards will be accepted the following year at RUSVM, and the undergraduate institution agrees to grant its baccalaureate degree to students who successfully complete the first two academic semesters at RUSVM. The undergraduate institution will have the sole discretion to determine the field of study in which the baccalaureate degree is awarded.

Royal Veterinary College, University of London

Margaret Kilyon
Head of Admissions
Royal Veterinary College
Royal College Street
London
NW1 0TU
UK
Telephone: (+44) 20 7468 5146
Fax: +44 (0)20 7388 2342
Email: international@rvc.ac.uk

The RVC has a successful record of training North American students and can count several hundred American and Canadian graduates as alumni. Founded in 1791, the RVC was the first veterinary school in the UK, and the driving force behind the establishment of the nation's veterinary profession. The first four students were admitted in January 1792, and ever since the College has been at the forefront of teaching and research in veterinary and allied sciences. The RVC was the first Veterinary School to submit a woman for membership to the Royal College of Veterinary Surgeons; become an independent veterinary school within a federal university; be accredited by the American Veterinary Medical Association; introduce a degree in Veterinary Nursing; and establish a Centre for Lifelong and Independent Veterinary Education. Today, first-class teaching and research staff, experienced in a wide range of disciplines and skills, help talented students to exploit state-of-the-art clinical facilities and laboratories to the full—maintaining the RVC's long, proud tradition of making seminal contributions to both the animal and human sciences.

We have one campus near Kings Cross/Camden Town, in central London (the London Campus) and one located close to the outskirts of London on a 575-acre site near Potters Bar (the Hertfordshire Campus). Both offer a friendly and supportive environment and excellent facilities for teaching and learning. The London Campus boasts newly refurbished research laboratories, and extensive library, an anatomy museum, the London Bioscience Innovation Centre and the Beaumont-Sainsbury Animal Hospital. Accommodation, a fitness room, a refectory and a bar, and a new social learning space including a café/deli are also on site and the clubs, bars, restaurants and theatres of Camden and London's West End are easily accessed on foot or by public transport. A twenty-minute walk from the London Campus is the University of London whose collegiate structure incorporates the RVC. Here in the capital's "university quarter," you will find some of the nation's greatest educational and research facilities. The Hertfordshire Campus is our main clinical campus with three state-of-the-art teaching hospitals on site including the largest veterinary-referral hospital in Europe. Located in rural countryside near Potters Bar, it is a 20 minute train journey from London's King's Cross station and comprises lecture theatres, laboratories, a Learning Resources Centre (providing superb IT resources and teaching and library facilities), a Clinical Skills Centre and student housing. There is also a refectory, sports fields, and a student-run bar. In addition to the modern journals and textbooks you will find in our libraries, the RVC has one of the best collections of old veterinary books in the world. The RVC has invested heavily in the Hertfordshire Campus in recent years, developing a new Student Village with over 190 bedrooms, a new refectory for both staff and students, a state-of-the-art Teaching and Research Centre and a world-class Equine Hospital. Our working-farm is also located at this campus.

Places in RVC halls of residence are available and students from overseas are given priority. The College has a number of dedicated staff who provide academic and pastoral support to students throughout the course, and we have an active and welcoming student community.

Application Information

For specific application information (availability, deadlines, fees and VM-CAS participation), please refer to our website at http://www.rvc.ac.uk/Undergraduate/International/Country/NorthAmerica.cfm.

Residency implications: The UK government introduced a points-based immigration system for students from non-EU countries who wish to study in the UK. For further information on entry to the UK, please refer to http://www.ukvisas.gov.uk/en/ and to the College's web site. Students must also be able to ensure adequate financial support for the duration of their course.

Prerequisites for Admission

Course requirements

VMCAS applicants are normally final year or recent university graduates although students with two years pre-vet will be considered. We will also consider High School students studying AP or the International Baccalaureate. These students apply through UCAS (see our website at http://www.rvc.ac.uk/Undergraduate/International/Country/NorthAmerica.cfm#Applying).   Science graduates or applicants in the final year of a science based degree with the prerequisites may be considered for our 4 year accelerated course. Applicants who are unsuccessful in gaining a place on the four year programme may be considered for our five year programme. Subjects must include Organic Chemistry with lab, Biochemistry, Mathematics or Statistics, Principles of Biology, Physics with lab, General Biology, and Animal Biology or Zoology all with lab. As a minimum we require 8 Upper Level semester credits in Organic

Chemistry and 8 Upper Level semester credits in Principles of Biology, General Biology, Animal Biology or Zoology and 4 semester credits in each of Biochemistry, Physics with Laboratory and Mathematics/Statistics (Algebra is acceptable). It is also recommended that students take General Chemistry or Fundamentals of Chemistry.

Required undergraduate GPA: 3.40 or higher preferred (on 4.0 point scale).

AP credit policy: not applicable for graduate applicants.

Course completion deadline: all required courses should be completed by July of the year of admission.

Standardized examinations: GRE General test required. RVC institution code is 3207.

Additional requirements and considerations
Applicants are also expected to have gained significant relevant work experience of handling animals. This should include work in veterinary practice and where possible other animal establishments.

Supplemental Application: Not required

Summary of Admission Procedure

Timetable
> VMCAS application deadline: Wednesday, October 2, 2013 at 1:00 p.m. Eastern Time
> Immediate offers which do not require an interview are made to exceptional candidates: October/November
> Interview dates are arranged: October-December
> Date interviews are held: January/February (held in the U.S.). Some interviews may be held earlier
> Date acceptances mailed: March/April (some may be sent earlier)
> School begins: September

Transcripts: All transcripts to VMCAS by 1 September 2013 and fall transcripts to VMCAS by 1 February 2014

Deposit (to hold place in class): £1,000 sterling

Deferments: may be considered in exceptional circumstances.

Evaluation criteria
> Academic performance
> Animal/veterinary experience
> Interview (in most cases)

References/evaluations (minimum 2 required—one from academic
science source and one from a veterinary surgeon who you have
worked with)
Personal statement

2011–2012 admissions summary (for entry in 2012)

	Number of Applicants	Number of New Entrants
In-province	1,098	186
International	432	44
Total:	1,530	230

Expenses for the 2012–2013 Academic Year*

Tuition and fees

Resident	residents of the UK are government-funded by loans
International	£20,300 sterling

Living Expenses

estimated living expenses given below represent a guide to the sum
required to live in reasonable comfort in London.

Single student: £10,555

Couples: £16,178 (plus an additional £2,000 per child)

* For up-to-date information on fees and all further information regarding admission to the College, please visit our website.

University of Saskatchewan-Western College of Veterinary Medicine

Admissions Office
Western College of Veterinary Medicine
52 Campus Drive
University of Saskatchewan
Saskatoon Saskatchewan S7N 5B4
Canada
Telephone: (306) 966-7459
www.usask.ca/wcvm

The Western College of Veterinary Medicine is located in the city of Saskatoon, which has a population of about 265,000 and is the major urban center in central Saskatchewan. The city is also the major commercial center for central and northern Saskatchewan and is served by 2 national airlines with direct connections to all major centers in Canada.

The Western College of Veterinary Medicine is one of the few veterinary colleges where all health sciences and agriculture are offered on the same campus. The college is devoted to undergraduate education and has a reputation in Canada and in the northwestern United States for educating veterinarians who are well-rounded in general veterinary medicine and have good practical backgrounds. It has one of the best field-service caseloads in North America.

Application Information

For specific application information (availability, deadlines, fees, and VMCAS participation), please refer to the contact information listed above.

Residency implications: Currently, 78 students are selected for quota positions from Alberta, British Columbia, Manitoba, Saskatchewan, and the Yukon, Nunavut, and Northwest Territories. Special consideration is given to self-identified individuals of aboriginal origin. Residents of foreign countries are not considered.

Prerequisites for Admission

Course requirements and semester hours

English	6
Physics	3
Biology	6
Genetics	3
Introductory chemistry	6
Organic chemistry	3

Mathematics or statistics	6
Biochemistry	3
Microbiology	3
Electives	21

Required undergraduate GPA: a minimum cumulative average of 75% is required.

Course completion deadline: prerequisite courses must be completed by the time of entry into the program.

Standardized examinations: none required.

Reference Forms: Two required - one from a veterinarian and one from an individual with an agricultural- or animal-related background.

Additional Requirements/Information: Space is provided on the application form to nominate referees to support the application. Referees will be contacted directly and asked to complete the reference form online.

Additional requirements and considerations
    Animal/veterinary work experience, motivation, and knowledge
    Maturity
    Leadership
    Communication skills

Summary of Admission Procedure

Timetable
    Application deadline: December 1
    Reference deadline: February 15
    Date interviews are held: May–June
    Date acceptances mailed: on or before July 1
    School begins: late August

Deposit (to hold place in class): none required.

Deferments: not considered.

Evaluation criteria
The 3-part admission procedure consists of an assessment of academic ability, a personal interview, and an overall assessment of the application file.

	% weight
Grades	60
Interview*	40

* Interview selection is based entirely on academic performance.

2012–2013 admissions summary

	Number of Applicants	*Number of New Entrants*
Resident	56	20
Contract[†]	282	57
Nonresident	2	2
Total:	340	79

Expenses for the 2012–2013 Academic Year

Tuition and fees

Resident	$8.254.06 $C
Nonresident	
Contract student[†]	$8,254.06 $C
Other nonresident-Canadian	$8,254.06 $C

† For further information, see the listing of contracting states and provinces.

St. George's University

Office of Admission
St. George's University
c/o The North American Correspondent
University Support Services, LLC
3500 Sunrise Highway
Building 300
Great River, NY 11739
Phone +1 (631) 665-8500, ext 91218
US/Canada Toll-Free 1(800) 899-6337, ext 9 1218
UK Free Phone: 0800 1699061
Fax: +1 (631) 665-5590
E-mail: SGUEnrolment@sgu.edu
Website: www.sgu.edu

Having received full accreditation by the AVMA COE in 2011, St. George's University School of Veterinary Medicine is proud of its academic excellence exemplified by its breadth of highly regarded education, unprecedented student support services, and internationally recognized faculty. The core mission of the University is creating excellent academic programs within an international setting where students and faculty are actively recruited from around the world. St. George's University has drawn faculty and students from over 140 countries, assembling a diverse community of disparate cultural and educational backgrounds.

Located on the southwest corner of the Caribbean island of Grenada, SGU's shoreline location offers its growing student body a serene environment in which to live, learn and create a worldwide network of friends and colleagues. Along with SGU's state-of-the-art facilities, complete with a large animal facility, marine station, and the SGU Small Animal Clinic, St. George's University School of Veterinary Medicine prepares its students for leadership, life-long success and service in a constantly changing world.

Over 6,000 students from throughout the world are enrolled in one of the three University's Schools: Medicine, Veterinary Medicine, and Arts and Sciences. SGU students also benefit from world-renowned international academic partnerships with universities, hospitals and other educational and scientific institutions.

The veterinary medical program is delivered with a number of entry options: the seven-, six- and five-year programs which begin with the preveterinary medical sciences and an option to enter directly into the four-year veterinary medical program. This enables students flexible entry points depending upon their academic backgrounds. Students accepted into the preveterinary medical sciences are placed in the appropriate program option (either the seven-, six- or five-year program track) according to their academic background and are enrolled in the veterinary medical program for five to seven years. Applicants accepted directly into the veterinary medical sciences generally complete the program in four years.

The DVM program is conducted on the University's main campus on the True Blue peninsula of Grenada, West Indies, except for the final year which is the clinical year spent at an affiliated AVMA-accredited School of Veterinary Medicine. These schools are located in the United States, Canada, United Kingdom, Ireland, and Australia.

Prerequisites for Admission

The requirements for direct entry into the four-year DVM program vary depending on the educational system of your home country. What is required for all applicants is completion of secondary school, a period of farm experience or time spent in a veterinary practice, and possession of a bachelor's degree from an accredited University or 60 credit hours.

The following specific undergraduate coursework (or its equivalent) is required as part of the preveterinary medical sciences requirements for admission (credit hours):

One year: General Biology or Zoology with lab (8)
One year: Inorganic Chemistry (General or Physical) with lab (8)
One semester: Organic Chemistry with lab (4)
One semester: Biochemistry (3)
One semester: Genetics (3)
One semester: Physics with lab (4)
One semester: Calculus, Computer Science or Statistics (3)
One semester: English (3)

Applicants from North America

A completed bachelor's degree from an accredited university or 90 credit hours is required for direct entry into the four-year veterinary medical program. A candidate may apply before completion of the bachelor's degree.

Standardized Examination: Candidates must submit scores by the corresponding application deadlines (see below) on the Graduate Record Examination or alternatively on the MCAT. (Our GRE Code is 7153; MCAT code 21303.)

A minimum of two and maximum of five letters of recommendation, (preferably from veterinarians or science professors) or a preveterinary medical committee evaluation, are required.

Applicants from the British System of Education

For direct entry into the four-year DVM program, a bachelor's degree with a strong science background is required.

Applicants with passes at the Advanced Level of the General Certificate of Education will be assessed individually and will be considered for appropriate entry into the five-year DVM program. Generally, A Level students with the appropriate courses and grades matriculate into the five-year veterinary medical program.

If English is not the principal language, the applicant must have achieved a score in the Test of English as a Foreign Language (TOEFL) of at least 600 points (written) or 250 points (computer-based).

Applicants from Other Systems of Education

An applicant must have achieved the successful completion of secondary school (twelve years post-kindergarten, comprising four years post-primary/ elementary, that, in itself is at least eight years long), preferably in a science curriculum or track.

An applicant must have completed a bachelor's degree (or its equivalent), which includes a science background and the study of English.

If English is not the principal language, the applicant must have achieved a score in the Test of English as a Foreign Language (TOEFL) of at least 600 points (written) or 250 points (computer-based).

Applicants who do not meet the admission requirements for direct entry into the four-year DVM program may apply for admission to either the seven-, six-, or five-year veterinary medical program that begin with the preveterinary medical sciences. Depending on the country of origin and academic background, a student enters the preveterinary medical sciences for a period of one to three years, with the full veterinary program ranging from four to seven years, depending upon the individual's point of entry.

Application Deadlines for August and January Matriculation

The School of Veterinary Medicine begins first-term classes in mid-August and again in mid-January. The Committee on Admission utilizes a rolling admission policy in the School of Veterinary Medicine; therefore, applications are accepted and reviewed on an ongoing basis. For students applying directly with the University, the final deadline for receipt of applications and all supporting documentation is June 15th of the current year for the August class and November 15th of the preceding year for the January class. For students applying using VMCAS, the application deadline is posted on the VMCAS application website.

Prospective candidates should note that entering classes are highly competitive and applications completed early have the advantage of being reviewed at the beginning of the admission's process.

The time necessary to secure official transcripts, standardized test scores and letters of recommendation should be taken into consideration. The Committee reserves the right to defer an application to the following semester if there are no available seats.

Interview:

The Office of Admission encourages candidates who have been approved for an interview to request interviews in Grenada and will schedule one upon the applicant's request. The University recognizes that financial considerations may prevent many candidates who reside at great distances from Grenada from choosing this option. Interviews, therefore, may be conducted in the United States, the United Kingdom, Africa, the Middle East, the Far East, the Caribbean or other locations that best serve the diverse applicant pool. Interviews are conducted by faculty members, visiting professors, or graduates of St. George's University and are mandatory for acceptance into the veterinary medical program.

Candidates are advised that being granted an interview is no guarantee of acceptance.

2012 admissions summary

January 2012 incoming class:

Total Applicants:	158	Entering Students:	61
US Applicants	132	US Applicants	52
Non-US	26	Non-US	9

August 2012 incoming class:

Total Applicants:	411	Entering Students:	105
US Applicants	347	US Applicants	93
Non-US	64	Non-US	12

Tuition and Fees are the same for all DVM students regardless of residence:
Years 1-3 (nonclinical years in Grenada) $33,368 yearly
Year 4 (clinical year at affiliated university) $59,202

Dual Degree Programs:

Combined DVM / MPH, MSc, and MBA degree programs are available.

Applications can be submitted online directly through the SGU website at www.sgu.edu or via the VMCAS application system. If you have questions about the application process, please call one of our admission advisors at 1 (800) 899-6337, ext 9 1280.

University of Sydney

Faculty of Veterinary Science
JD Stewart building
University of Sydney
Sydney NSW 2006
Telephone: 02 9351 2441
Fax: 02 9351 3056
Email: vet.science@sydney.edu.au
Website: http://sydney.edu.au/vetscience

The University of Sydney, founded in 1850, is Australia's first university. Over the past 150 years, the University has built an international reputation for its outstanding teaching and as a centre of research excellence. It is one of the largest universities in Australia, with over 47,000 students, including 9,000 international students from more than 100 different countries. Famous for its sandstone buildings, lawns, courtyards and parklands setting the University of Sydney's main campus is spread across 72-hectares and features sports ovals, three sports centres, indoor and outdoor swimming pools, two major complexes devoted to student recreation and services, the famous Quadrangle and many other beautiful modern and historic buildings.

Located only ten minutes by bus from the heart of the Sydney business district, the main campus provides easy access to national and international companies based in the city and its surrounding suburbs.

The Faculty of Veterinary Science was established in 1910 and is the oldest continuing Faculty of its kind in Australia. The Faculty is an international leader in veterinary and animal education and research. The Faculty maintains teaching hospitals on both the Camperdown and Camden campuses, where students and veterinarians work together in a clinical teaching and learning environment. Referral and primary accession cases are seen at both sites, while the University Veterinary Teaching Hospital at Camden also provides veterinary services to farms in the region. A wide range of companion animals, farm animals, racing animals, exotic and native species are seen.

The Faculty delivers inspirational and innovative student-centred teaching that leads to an acceptance of the need for life-long, evidence-based learning whilst also providing clinical and research excellence through creative, collaborative programs.

The Veterinary Science program produces graduates with the knowledge and skills to pursue many career options as veterinary scientists participating in the care and welfare of animals. Completion of the course ensures students have a wide knowledge of the principles associated with every aspect of health and disease in animals – domestic and native.

Entry Pathways

In 2015 the University of Sydney will be moving to a four-year graduate entry Doctor of Veterinary Medicine (DVM). Students will be able to enter the program by two pathways:

1. **Undergraduate applicants:** From 2014 students can apply for entry into a combined six-year degree program commencing with a Bachelor of Veterinary Biology (BVetBiol) and on the successful completion of the first two years will be eligible to progress to the Veterinary Medicine program.

   Prerequisites

   Admission to the BVetBiol is based on a level of assumed knowledge, comprising Higher School Certificate (HSC) (or equivalent) chemistry, mathematics and physics, with biology as a distinct advantage. Prospective students who have not reached this level in these subjects will be permitted to enrol but must be aware of the need to undertake supplementary work to avoid placing themselves at a disadvantage.

2. **Graduate applicants:** Students may also complete a science based bachelor degree from Sydney or any other institution and then apply for entry into year one of the DVM program which will be available from 2015.

   Prerequisites

   Students will need to have successfully completed at least one semester of study in general chemistry (physical and inorganic), organic chemistry, biology and biochemistry as part of their science degree.

Admission Requirements

Academic Performance: International students must have achieved a similar standard to that expected of an Australian student seeking entry. Applicants will be assessed on the basis of their academic achievement in their final year of secondary education (Year 12 or equivalent) for the BVetBiol or their tertiary studies from a recognized University for entry into the DVM. Minimum GPA required for DVM entry is 3.00 on a 4.00 scale, however, applicants must demonstrate and aptitude for the sciences.

Standardized examinations: Direct entry into the DVM requires students to submit result from the International Student Admission Test (ISAT) http://www.acer.edu.au/isat (Applicants may submit GRE scores in lieu of ISAT scores.)

Additional requirements and considerations: All applicants are expected to have gained relevant work experience and animal handling. This should be demonstrated on the "Commitment to Veterinary Science" form that can be downloaded from the faculty web site http://sydney.edu.au/vetscience/future students/

Practical Experience

During the inter-semester and intra-semester breaks students are required to undertake, placements for preparatory clinical experience and animal husbandry. The final year is lecture free with students participating in practice-based activities and the management and care of patients.

Professional Recognition

Sydney graduates are immediately eligible for registration for practice by all Australian state and territory veterinary surgeons' boards and are recognised by the Royal College of Veterinary Surgeons in the United Kingdom and the American Veterinary Medical Association.

Additional Information

Application deadline: 31 October, however late applications will be considered if the quota has not been reached. Applications will be accepted throughout the year and assessed as soon as they are received.

Standardize Test deadline: 31 October. Results must be submitted with application.

All international applicants must apply directly to the University of Sydney International Office using the On-line Application system. http://sydney.edu.au/internationaloffice/forms/index.shtml.

For more information please visit the International Office website at http://sydney.edu.au/internationaloffice/.

New Entrants

Australian resident	90
International	40

Tuition Fees 2013

International Student	AUD$49,920
Australian resident (government supported)	AUD$9,792
Australian resident	AUD$45,120

Tuition fees are indexed annually.

Utrecht University[*]

Office for International Cooperation
Faculty of Veterinary Medicine
Utrecht University
Yalelaan 1
3584 CL Utrecht
The Netherlands
Telephone: +31.30.2532116
Email: bic@vet.uu.nl
www.uu.nl/vct

Short history

In 1821 a state veterinary school was founded in Utrecht. Almost a century later, in 1918, the school acquired the status of an institution of higher learning and in 1925 it was incorporated into the State University of Utrecht and thereby became the first and until to date the only Faculty of Veterinary Medicine in the Netherlands. Utrecht University, founded in 1636, is one of the 14 universities in the Netherlands. The faculty of Veterinary Medicine is now one of the 6 faculties of Utrecht University and is located at campus site De Uithof just outside the city of Utrecht. The Faculty of Veterinary Medicine is housed in modern and spacious buildings on a total surface of 60.000 m).

Organisation and staff

The faculty encompasses 8 departments with specialized facilities, a Faculty Office and a number of general services (e.g. leaning environment with audio-visual units and the library, pharmacy, experimental farms, museum, student computer rooms etc). The faculty has an academic staff of 418 fte, including 32 full professors and an administrative and support staff of 484 fte. Most staff members can communicate well in English and most lecturers have experience in teaching veterinary medicine in the English language.

Veterinary education

Admission of students to the 6-year veterinary training programme (taught in Dutch) is limited to 225 each year, resulting in a total of 1400 students. The veterinary curriculum leads to the "dierenarts' degree (Doctor of Veterinary Medicine, DVM). In September 2007 the veterinary education under a Bachelor - Master (3+3 years) structure started with the 1st year of the bachelor programme.

[*] These pages are for last year's admissions cycle (2012-2013). For updated information, please visit: http://www.uu.nl/university/international-students/EN/admission/Pages/default.aspx

Research and postgraduate education

Research at the faculty of Veterinary Medicine is the responsibility of the Institute for Veterinary Research (IVR). Research which is conducted as part of the postgraduate master programmes and PhD programme is linked to one of the research programmes of the IVR. The postgraduate master programmes were initiated from 1994 onwards and are now integrated in the postgraduate educational Master of Science programme Veterinary Science.

Quality of education

The faculty of Veterinary Medicine is accredited by the American Veterinary Medical Association (AVMA) and Canadian Veterinary Medical Association (CVMA) since 1973, the European Association of Establishments of Veterinary Education and the Dutch and Flemish Accreditation Organization.

Information about the admission to the Faculty of Veterinary Medicine for foreign students

Special rules apply for the study of Veterinary Medicine. The Dutch Ministry of Education has declared the so-called numerus fixus applicable to the study of Veterinary Medicine. This entails that only a limited amount of students is admitted each year. The number of admission requests largely exceeds the number of allocations. Those restrictions affect both Dutch and foreign students. The available places are assigned by selection through interviews or drawing lots.

Application and Drawing Lots

Each year the minister of Education and Science determines the number of students that can be admitted to the study of Veterinary Medicine. At this moment the number is 225. In order to take part in the lottery for placement, you need to complete an application form via Internet (start with website: www. uu.nl) and send this in before May 15th.

If you do not apply you cannot participate in drawing lots.

Foreign diplomas

Foreign diplomas have to be evaluated and compared with the Dutch equivalent diplomas. This evaluation takes time and can result in the fact that you have to take supplementary exams before being accepted for the lottery.

Information about the evaluation of your diplomas can be obtained at:
Universiteit Utrecht, Admissions Office
P.O. Box 80 125, 3508 TC Utrecht, the Netherlands
Phone: +31 30 253 7000
Visiting Address: Leuvenlaan 19, Utrecht – De Uithof

Dutch Language Exam

If the result of the lottery is favorable, then - prior to admission to the study of Veterinary Medicine - you have to prove your (sufficient) knowledge of the Dutch language. This is a requirement under the Dutch law because the education is in the Dutch language. The owner of a foreign diploma therefore has to pass the exam "Dutch as Second Language program 2" (*Staatsexamen Nederlands als Tweede Taal, programma 2*) before being admitted.

Request information about language courses and the examinations at:
James Boswell Institute
P.O. Box 80148, 3508 TC Utrecht, The Netherlands
Phone: +31 30 253 8666

Tuition fees and scholarships

The tuition fee depends on your nationality and the programme you register for:

Nationality	Programme	Tuition 2012-2013
EU / EEA	Bachelor's and Master's programmes	€1,771
Non EU / EEA	Bachelor Veterinary Medicine	€10,500
	Master Veterinary Medicine	€19,500

No financial aid is offered to foreign students. Neither the government nor the university grants scholarships to foreign students.

Residence Permit

Every foreign student who wants to receive academic education in the Netherlands needs a residence permit. More information can be obtained at the Admissions Office.

Documentation

When requesting admission, the following pieces of documentation have to be sent to the Admissions Office (see above):

- a short and concise curriculum vitae with a complete overview of the education
- a certified copy of the birth register
- certified copies of diplomas, subject overview, list of marks of secondary and (pre-) university education in Dutch, French, German, or English
- a copy of personal details from the passport

For further information about the admission to the study of Veterinary Medicine please contact:

Student advisor
Faculty of Veterinary Medicine
Department of Educational and Student Affairs/Office for International Cooperation
PO Box 80 163, 3508 TD Utrecht, the Netherlands
e-mail: osz@vet.uu.nl

AAVMC Affiliate Member Veterinary Medical Schools

Non-AVMA / COE Accredited

University of Copenhagen

Office for International Cooperation
Faculty of Health and Medical Sciences
University of Copenhagen
Blegdamsvej 3B
DK-2200 København N
Denmark
Telephone: +45 35 33 35 89
Email: hhd@sund.ku.dk
www.sund.ku.dk

Short history

The Veterinary School in Copenhagen was founded in 1773 as one of the first schools in the world. In 1856 the veterinary school was moved to its present location and at that time acquired the status of an institution of higher learning incorporating agriculture and animal science. In 2007 the Royal Veterinary and Agricultural University merged with the University of Copenhagen and was transformed into the Faculty of Life Sciences incorporating the veterinary school. The University of Copenhagen was inaugurated on 1 June 1479, after King Christian I was granted approval for its establishment by Pope Sixtus IV. Based on a German model, the university consisted of four faculties: Theology, Law, Medicine and Philosophy. Today with more than 37,000 students and more than 7,000 employees, the University of Copenhagen is the largest institution of research and education in Denmark. The purpose of the University – to quote the University Statute – is to 'conduct research and provide further education to the highest academic level'.

Approximately one hundred different institutes, departments, laboratories, centers, museums, etc., form the nucleus of the University, where professors, lecturers and other academic staff, as well as most of the technical and administrative personnel, carry out their daily work, and where teaching takes place. With the opening of the totally rebuilt and modernized Small Animal University Hospital at the Frederiksberg Campus in early 2011 the Copenhagen Veterinary School including the newly built Large Animal University Hospital at the Taastrup Campus functions as one of the most modern veterinary schools with state of the art equipment.

In January 2012 the Copenhagen School of Veterinary Medicine and Animal Science merged with the Faculty of Pharmaceutical Sciences and the Faculty of Health to form a new, scientifically and financially strong Faculty of Health and Medicine within the University of Copenhagen.

Organisation and staff

The veterinary school encompasses 3 departments with specialized facilities, a Faculty Office and a number of general services (e.g. learning environment 204 with audio-visual units, library, pharmacy, experimental farms, student facilities including several computer rooms etc). The veterinary school has an academic staff of 154 fte, including 29 full professors and an administrative and support staff of 221 fte. Most staff members communicate well in English and most faculties have experience in teaching veterinary medicine in English. In early 2012 all faculty have completed officially approved proficiency tests in English.

Undergraduate veterinary education

Admission of students to the 5½-year undergraduate veterinary training programme is limited to 180 each year, resulting in a total of 1100 students. They pass full examinations at the completion of each course.

Research and postgraduate education

Research at Faculty of Health and Medical Sciences is the responsibility of the Vice Dean for Research and the department heads. Research which is conducted as part of the PhD programmes is included in this portfolio.

Quality of education

The School of Veterinary Medicine and Animal Sciences has been regularly evaluated and accredited by the European Association of Establishments of Veterinary Education since 1988 (latest accreditation in 2010) and had a pre Site Visit by the American Veterinary Medical Association (AVMA) in 2009. A full site visit is expected to be applied for in 2013.

Information about the admission to the Faculty of Veterinary Medicine for foreign students

In general foreign students have access to the Danish universities. Non-EU citizens must apply for visa before being allowed to apply.

Special rules apply for the study of Veterinary Medicine. The Danish Ministry of Science has declared a numerus clausus to the DVM programme. This entails that only a limited amount of students is admitted each year. The number of admission requests largely exceeds the number of allocations. Restrictions affect both Danish and foreign students. The available places are assigned by selection through interviews (50%) or based upon grades obtained in high school (50%). Letters of recommendation are neither required nor accepted.

Application to the Danish DVM program

Each year the minister of education and science lays down the number of students to be admitted to the DVM programme. Currently 180 students are accepted in each class. There are two routes of application. The first is solely based upon high school grades (Quota I) and the second is based upon a mixture of high school grades, a written admission test, and an interview, in which work experience, motivation, and knowledge of animals and the veterinary profession are weighted highly (Quota II). Application deadline for Quota I is 5 July 2013, and for Quota II the application deadline is 15 March 2013.

International students are referred to http://studier.ku.dk/internationalstudents/ for further information about application for the DVM programme.

Tuition fees and scholarships

Generally students from within the European Union do not pay tuition fee. For foreign students please refer to web site of the Ministry of Science, Technology and Innovation http://en.vtu.dk/.

Generally financial aid is not offered to foreign students.

Residence permit

Foreign students who want to receive an academic education in Denmark need a residence permit. More information can be obtained at the Office for International Cooperation or at a Danish embassy in the country of origin.

Additionally applicants must demonstrate access to sufficient financial means. The amount varies and more detailed information should be sought at a Danish embassy.

St. Matthew's University

School of Veterinary Medicine
Campus:
P.O. Box 32330
Grand Cayman KY1-1209
CAYMAN ISLANDS
Telephone: 345-745-3199

Administrative Office:
12124 High Tech Ave., Suite 350
Orlando, FL 32817
Telephone: 800.498.9700
Email: admissions@stmatthews.edu
www.stmatthews.edu

St. Matthew's University School of Veterinary Medicine is located on beautiful Grand Cayman in the Caribbean. Grand Cayman is the fifth largest financial district in the world and has a highly developed infrastructure which is very comparable to the United States. It is also one of the safest islands in the Caribbean, boasting one of the lowest crime and poverty rates. Grand Cayman has hundreds of restaurants, scores of banks, world-class hotels, and many opportunities for boating, diving, horseback riding, and other recreation. The island is less than an hour's flight from Miami, and also has direct flights from Atlanta, Chicago, Charlotte, Houston, Tampa, Toronto, Washington D.C., and other locations.

At SMU, we are as committed to your dreams as you are. Throughout your ten semesters with us, we will do everything we can to ensure your success by supporting all aspects of your education and life, including:

Focus on Teaching: Dedicated, talented faculty whose time commitments are focused on teaching and mentoring.

Student Mentors: Student mentors understand about adjusting to life in veterinary school, and are eager to see you succeed.

Very Low Student to Faculty Ratio: With a student to faculty ratio of less than five to one, you will have an unprecedented level of faculty support and attention. We limit each incoming cohort of students to a maximum of 35.

Best Value: Most affordable tuition of any Caribbean veterinary school.

Accelerated Schedule: Complete your pre-clinical education on Grand Cayman in just 28 months, and then return to the U.S. or Canada for clinical training, with the ability to complete vet school in just over three years.

SMU's modern, state-of-the-art main campus is located across the street from beautiful Seven Mile Beach, and boasts wireless technology throughout the bright, air-conditioned classrooms, labs, library, and student lounges. SMU also has a new clinical Teaching Facility which hosts surgery, medicine and clinical skills training as well as anatomy and pathology laboratories. Students have the opportunity to travel to local farms with veterinary staff from the Cayman Department of Agriculture. Presently, the students spend seven (7) semesters on Grand Cayman and their final 12 months in clinical programs at one of our many AVMA-accredited Clinical Program Affiliate Schools in the United States and Canada.

There are significant opportunities for students to gain experience with exotic species through our collaborations with the Cayman Turtle Farm, Central Caribbean Marine Institute, Dolphin Discovery, the Blue Iguana Project and the Coral Reef Research Program.

Application Information

We welcome applications from any qualified candidate who dreams of becoming a veterinarian. For specific application information (availability, deadlines, fees, transferring to SMU and VMCAS participation), please refer to the contact information listed above.

Prerequisites for Admission

Course Requirements and semester hours:

General Biology*	8
General Chemistry*	8
Organic Chemistry*	4
Biochemistry	3
Language Arts (English)	6
College Math or Computer Science	3
Physics (Recommended)	4
Social Science (Recommended)	6

These courses must include an attached laboratory.

Course completion deadline: all prerequisite courses must be completed prior to matriculation.

Standardized Examinations: Graduate Record Examination (GRE®), general test, is not required but is strongly recommended. The exam must have been taken within the previous five calendar years, and scores must be sent to the Office of Admissions as part of the application for admission.

Additional Considerations: Each candidate is carefully evaluated on the basis of these factors:

Academic background
Overall grade point average
Science grade point average
Strength of major/minor
GRE scores
2 Letters of Reference (electronic or written; one should be from a veterinarian)
Personal statement
College activities that demonstrate service to the community
Personal Interview (by invitation)

Summary of Admission Procedure

Timetable
> Application deadlines: None. Rolling admissions. Three incoming cohorts per year.
> Interviews: Held in person or via telephone/videoconference.
> Acceptance notification: Within two weeks of interview.
> School begins: August, January, May (three start dates per year).

Deposit (to hold place in class): $500.00

Deferments: Considered on an individual basis.

Evaluation criteria: The 3-part admission procedure includes an objective evaluation of academic credentials, a subjective review of personal credentials and an interview by invitation.

Transfer: Transfer credits (advanced standing) may be awarded at the discretion of the University. No transfers are permitted later than beginning of Semester 5.

Seats generally available: Maximum of 35 (total) seats available per incoming cohort to ensure exceptional level of faculty support for students.

Expenses for the 2012–2013 Academic Year

Tuition and fees

Pre-Clinical Sciences (Grand Cayman)	$10,875
Clinical Sciences (Clinical Affiliates)	$17,700
Additional fees	$275

Dual-Degree Programs

MBA graduate degree program is available.
Visit our site at http://www.stmatthews.edu/vet_curriculum_concurrent-degree-program.shtml

POLICIES ON ADVANCED STANDING

Transfers are permitted to most colleges of veterinary medicine in the United States under specified conditions. Typical requirements include a vacancy in the class, completion of all prerequisite requirements, and compatible curricula. Following is a listing of schools and some of the conditions under which they will consider a transfer from another veterinary college with advanced standing. More detailed information may be obtained by writing to the individual schools in which you have an interest.

UNITED STATES

University of California, Davis

Applications may be considered if available positions exist within the third-year classes. Currently, each class in the DVM program of the School of Veterinary Medicine shall consist of no more than 138 students.

1. The applicant must have a strong academic record in his/her undergraduate program.
2. The applicant must be currently enrolled in an AVMA-accredited DVM program and must be in excellent academic and ethical standing in that program. The specific minimum benchmark will be that the applicant is in the top quartile of students in the Veterinary School in which the applicant is currently enrolled as determined by GPA or class rank.
3. The applicant must have completed veterinary course work equivalent to that expected of the students in the DVM program of the School of Veterinary Medicine, UC Davis, who will be in the same academic class.
4. The applicant has a valid reason for requesting admission in advanced standing.

University of Florida

1. An opening must exist in the second- or third-year class.
2. Students are only rarely considered for advanced standing based on exceptional personal circumstances.
3. Student must be enrolled in an AVMA accredited college.
4. Student must meet all prerequisites for admission as a first-year student (including GRE® scores).
5. The curricula of the two schools must be sufficiently alike to allow a student to enter without deficiencies in academic background.
6. Applicants must have a letter approving transfer from their dean or associate dean.

University of Georgia

1. Priority is given to Georgia residents, followed by contract state residents, then all other applicants.
2. Applicants will be considered for entry into the DVM degree program up to the third year of the curriculum, when and if space is available, as defined by the Admissions Committee.
3. Applications must include official transcripts of all completed veterinary and pre-veterinary coursework and a letter of support written by a senior administrator of the school in which the applicant is currently enrolled stating the applicant is currently in good academic standing.
4. No individual is eligible for transfer who has been dismissed or is on probation at any other school or college for deficiency in scholarship or because of misconduct.

University of Illinois

1. Transfer students will only be considered for the beginning of the second year of veterinary medicine and only if transfer seats become available in that class.
2. All prerequisite science courses must be completed prior to the request for transfer.
3. Minimum grade requirements include:
   cumulative and science GPAs of 2.75 on a 4.00 scale (doesn't include veterinary work);
   results of the Graduate Record Examination General Test completed within the last two years.
4. Student must complete the same preveterinary coursework as required for students accepted to the first year of the program.
5. Student must be in good academic standing.
6. To be considered for transfer, a student must present credentials for *preprofessional work* that fulfill the University of Illinois College of Veterinary Medicine requirements for first-year entry.
7. Complete information and an application can be found at vetmed.illinois.edu/asa/brochure.

Colorado State University

Transfer is dependent on position openings in the year into which the student transfers (most transfers will involve the loss of a year because of differences in school curricula). Candidate must:

1. have successfully completed at least the first year (equivalent of two semesters) of veterinary curriculum at an AVMA accredited college of veterinary medicine.

AND

2. have obtained the equivalent of a 3.0 cumulative GPA in your veterinary program AND must not have received a D, F, or unsatisfactory grade of any kind since enrolling in veterinary school.

AND

3. have a preveterinary academic record comparable to currently enrolled DVM students.

AND

4. provide evidence of noncognitive attributes comparable to currently enrolled DVM students.

If a veterinary student with an interest in transferring to CSU's DVM program meets ALL of the above minimum requirements, he/she may apply to the DVM program. To apply for transfer to CSU's Veterinary Program, please see http://www.cvmbs.colostate.edu/ns/_docs/students/dvm_policy_transfer_students.pdf.

Cornell University

1. Students are considered for advanced standing in rare and exceptional circumstances. Each request for transfer is considered on an individual basis.
2. Transfer students will be considered if an opening exists in the second-year class. Students seeking advanced standing may enter the DVM program at two points: at the beginning of the second year of study, or mid-way through the second year, at the beginning of the fourth (Spring) semester of study.
3. Students seeking advanced standing must be enrolled in an AVMA-accredited veterinary college.
4. The curricula of the two schools must be sufficiently similar to allow students to enter without deficiencies in their academic background.
5. Students must meet all *pre-veterinary* requirements for first-year entry at the College of Veterinary Medicine at Cornell University (including GRE scores, prerequisite coursework, animal and veterinary experience), and may not have any failing grades on their veterinary transcript.
6. Scores from the Graduate Record Examination (GRE) or Medical College Admissions Test (MCAT) may not be older than five years.
7. Applicants seeking advanced standing must include a letter from their Associate Dean certifying that the student is in good academic standing, has not been on academic probation, and has not been subject to any disciplinary action or dismissal for any reason.
8. Applicants are required to have completed at least two full semesters at the institution from which the transfer is requested. Only veterinary coursework completed at an AVMA-accredited institution will be considered.

9. After analyzing the academic background of the applicant, the Admissions Committee will place each accepted transfer student in the semester of study in the DVM curriculum deemed most appropriate. (*Veterinary course syllabi will be required at time of application*).

Iowa State University

Acceptance of students for advanced standing is on the recommendation of the Academic Standards Committee. Space must be available in the class to which the student is applying. See website, http://vetmed.iastate.edu/academics/prospective-students/admissions/transfer-admissions, for the transfer application form and further details.

Kansas State University

Acceptance of students for transfer is on recommendation of the Admissions Committee on a space-available basis.

Louisiana State University

1. There must be a vacancy in the class.
2. The curricula must be compatible.
3. The student must be in good academic standing with at least a 3.2 GPA in veterinary coursework at his/her present college.
4. Admission is limited to the second year of the program and only into the fall semester.
5. Each request for transfer is considered on a case-by-case basis.
6. To initiate the transfer process, please carefully read the DVM Transfer Guidelines information at www.vetmed.lsu.edu/admissions/transfer_apps.asp.

Michigan State University

1. Admission consideration is offered only to those current matriculants in professional veterinary curricula who believe that there are extenuating circumstances that would precipitate significant undue hardship if they continue at their current institution.
2. Applicants requesting a transfer must contact the Dean of Academic and Student Affairs at the school they are currently attending and notify him or her of their intent.
3. Applicants must also demonstrate quality academic performance throughout their professional school enrollment.
4. The curricula of the two schools must be sufficiently alike to allow a student to enter the second-year class without deficiencies in academic background.
5. All selection criteria for regular applicants apply to transfer applicants.

6. Priority is given to Michigan residents.
7. Applicants who have previously been denied admission to MSU CVM will not be considered for transfer admissions.
8. Space must be available.
9. AVMA accreditation of current school is considered.

University of Minnesota
1. Transfer students are accepted on a space available basis. The Admissions Committee will place each applicant in the year or semester of the curriculum deemed appropriate after analysis of equivalency of the required courses involved.
2. No academic work or standing will be accepted from DVM curricula other than those deemed accredited by the American Veterinary Medical Association.
3. All applicants must be U.S. citizens or holders of appropriate visas.
4. All applicants are required to have finished at least one full academic year at the institution from which transfer is requested and must be in good academic standing at the time of discontinuance according to written verification from the institution.
5. All applicants must have achieved a cumulative GPA of 3.00 (of 4.00) for the required courses at the initial institution.
6. Please visit the following website for more details: http://www.cvm.umn.edu/education/prospective/transferring/home.html

Mississippi State University

The Mississippi State University College of Veterinary Medicine accepts, on a limited basis, transfer students from other veterinary medical colleges to fill vacancies in the freshmen or sophomore classes. Transfer guidelines are as follows:

From a veterinary school not accredited by the AVMA:
Applicants for transfer into the second semester of the first year must have completed coursework equivalent to coursework taught in the first semester of the first year at MSU-CVM.

Applicants for transfer into the first semester of the second year must have completed coursework equivalent to coursework taught in the first year at MSU-CVM.

Applicants for transfer into the second semester of the second year must have completed coursework equivalent to all coursework taught in the first three semesters at MSU-CVM plus have had equivalent surgery laboratories.

From a veterinary school accredited by the AVMA:

Applicants are considered on a case-by-case basis with regard to length of time in current program.

General:

Any applicant considered for transfer admission must be in good academic standing (defined as being eligible to continue at current school from current point in the curriculum), never have failed a course while in veterinary medical school, never have been dismissed from a veterinary school and must have completed at least a full academic year at current veterinary school.

Any applicants considered for transfer admission will be required to attend an interview at Mississippi State University.

Typically, transfer applicants are not accepted into our program at a point later than first semester of the sophomore year. Accordingly, if a student should pursue application to Mississippi State University College of Veterinary Medicine and be accepted, it would be necessary for that student to complete at least two years at Mississippi State University to be eligible for a degree.

Students accepted for transfer are required to meet the current computer requirements of the college.

For more information, contact Tonya Calmes, Admissions Assistant, 662-325-4161, tcalmes@cvm.msstate.edu.

University of Missouri

1. Must be a vacancy in the class.
2. Will consider students who are U.S. citizens or holders of permanent alien visas and who have finished at least two years in a college of veterinary medicine that is AVMA accredited.
3. Students must be in good academic standing, never been denied admission from the University of Missouri for a first year position, and submit a letter of reference from the dean's office of the present college is required.

North Carolina State University

1. Must be a vacancy in the class.
2. Consideration by the Admission Committee on an individual basis.
3. Curricula must be compatible.
4. A letter from the dean of the current school certifying the applicant's academic standing.
5. Letter of recommendation from a faculty member at the original college.
6. Only accept transfers from AVMA accredited colleges.
7. At least 50% of DVM credit hours must be completed at North Carolina State in order to earn a North Carolina State University degree.

215

The Ohio State University

The Ohio State University does not accept transfer students.

Oklahoma State University

Transfer students are considered. Each application is evaluated on an individual basis. See website for transfer guide. http://www.cvhs.okstate.edu

Oregon State University

Admission of students with advanced standing is considered only in certain circumstances, and each case is considered on an individual basis.

University of Pennsylvania

PennVet does not consider transfer applications.

Purdue University

1. Positions must be available in the relevant class.
2. Student must be in good academic standing in his/her present program.
3. Students must have completed 1–2 years of DVM courses with an **exceptional** academic record in those courses.
4. Veterinary medical curricula must be compatible.
5. Student must have support of the administration from the program in which he/she is currently enrolled.

Please visit the following website for more specific detail: http://www.vet.purdue.edu/dvm/files/documents/transfer_policy.pdf

University of Tennessee

Admission of students with advanced standing (transfer) may be considered for unique circumstances on a case-by-case basis.

1. Position(s) must be available in the class into which one would like to matriculate.
2. Curricula of the two schools must be sufficiently alike to allow a student to matriculate without deficiencies in his/her academic background.
3. The applicant's academic dean must provide a letter approving transfer and indicating that the student is in good standing at his/her current college/school of veterinary medicine.
4. Admission is usually limited to the second semester of the first year of the DVM curriculum except for exceptional circumstances.
5. Letters of reference are required.

The Admissions Committee will review applicant credentials and interview those determined to best meet admission criteria.

Texas A & M University

Students requesting advanced standing must meet the following requirements:

1. Must have completed all previous professional veterinary courses in an AVMA accredited college of veterinary medicine.
2. Must have successfully completed the academic term preceding the semester into which student requests admission.
3. Must comply with all requirements for transfer into the university as described in the current catalog.
4. May request transfer only into the second through seventh semesters of the professional curriculum.
5. At the time of matriculation the student must certify by letter that he/she has not been convicted of crimes in the period from first enrollment in the college of veterinary medicine from which the student desires transfer until date of matriculation at Texas A&M University.
6. To request transfer consideration, the student must meet all requirements as posted on the College website at http://www.cvm.tamu.edu/dcvm/admissions/transferpol.shtml.

Tufts University

Applicants from other veterinary schools are considered. Students with advanced standing are admitted if and when space becomes available in the second-year class. The application deadline is June 1 for the following September. Please refer to our web site for details: http://www.tufts.edu/vet/

Tuskegee University

General: In most instances, transfer of a DVM student from their current program into the DVM program at Tuskegee will not be possible. However, in some cases transfer can be accomplished if a series of criteria can be met.

Criteria required for transfer: There are six specific criteria that must be met in order for a DVM student matriculating at another veterinary school or college of veterinary medicine to transfer into the DVM program at Tuskegee University School of Veterinary Medicine (TUSVM). These criteria are listed below.

1. The student seeking transfer to TUSVM must be currently enrolled in a school or college of veterinary medicine that is fully accredited by the American Veterinary Medical Association Counsel ob Education,
2. The student seeking to transfer to TUSVM must be in good academic standing at the veterinary school or college they are matriculating.
3. The DVM curriculum at the perspective transferees' school or college of matriculation must be sufficiently similar to the DVM curriculum at TUSVM to make transfer possible.

4. The perspective transferees' reason(s) for wanting to effect a transfer from their current DVM program to the DVM program at TUSVM must be evaluated and deemed an appropriate reason(s).
5. The perspective transferee must have either the Associate Dean For Academic Affairs or the Dean of their current DVM program submit a letter to the Director of Veterinary Admissions at TUSVM which specifically reaffirms the reason(s) for wanting to transfer and which also states that the perspective transferee is not under any present non-academic probationary status or under any present or pending disciplinary action(s).
6. The transfer must be approved by the Dean of the Tuskegee University College of Veterinary Medicine, Nursing, and Allied Health.

Virginia-Maryland Regional College of Veterinary Medicine

VMRCVM accepts students for advanced standing on the recommendation of the Admissions Committee on a space-available basis.

Washington State University

Admission of students with advanced standing is considered only in very specific and unique circumstances, and each case is considered on an individual basis.

University of Wisconsin

Wisconsin does not accept advanced standing students for admission.

INTERNATIONAL

Massey University

Applications for admission with advanced standing will only be considered by students enrolled in a veterinary program with a compatible curriculum, and pending an available space in the appropriate stage of the program. Applicants should contact vetschool@massey.ac.nz to apply for advanced standing.

Murdoch University

Applications for advanced standing will only be considered from students whose studies have been completed in a DVM program. Applicants are required to apply formally for advanced standing and provide the necessary documentation to allow for a full comparison between the previous study and Murdoch University's unit requirements. Prior courses must duplicate or substantially overlap multiple factors including breadth and depth of content, duration, objectives, assessment, context, and academic standard (level of intellectual effort required) for exemption to be granted.

St. Matthew's University

Applications for admission with advanced standing are welcomed from students from veterinary schools recognized by the American Veterinary Medical Association (AVMA) and/or the American Association of Veterinary State Boards (AAVSB). Transfer applicants must submit a complete application package to ensure a timely review. Acceptance of transfer credit is at the discretion of St. Matthew's University.

University of Calgary

Applications for admission to advanced semesters may be considered from students who have been enrolled in DVM programs at other institutions, subject to the availability of spaces in the DVM Program and the academic standing of the candidate. When places are available, candidates may be asked to present themselves for an interview and may be asked to pass examinations on subject matter in the veterinary curriculum. Applicants are advised that vacancies are rare and that restrictions on residency and citizenship status may be applied.

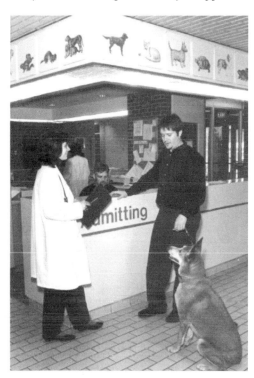

Small-animal care in a clinic is but one of many options for hands-on training at veterinary medical colleges. Photo courtesy of Atlantic Veterinary College, University of Prince Edward Island.

University of Prince Edward Island

Applicants who have completed all or portions of a veterinary medical program may apply for advanced standing to the second year of the DVM program.

Applicants for advanced standing must present evidence of educational accomplishments and may be required to address missing courses or competencies expected of our incoming second-year students. Students admitted with advanced standing must begin the college year in September.

The candidate must file a formal application and may be interviewed by the Admissions Committee and possibly other faculty. Places for admission to the college with advanced standing are limited and depend on vacancies.

It is imperative that the Admissions Committee have detailed and translated summaries of veterinary medical academic programs and accomplishments for those seeking advanced placement from schools in foreign countries.

Advanced-standing applications should be on file and completed as early as possible and no later than January 1. Candidates are strongly encouraged to visit the website http://www.upei.ca/programsandcourses/transfer-and-advanced-standing-applicants-dvm.

University of Queensland

Applications for advanced standing will only be considered from students whose studies have been completed in a veterinary program with a compatible curriculum, and where a space is available in the appropriate stage of the program. Please refer to the University of Queensland Policy 3.50.03 - Credit for Previous Studies and Recognised Prior Learning (http://ppl.app.uq.edu.au/) or contact the School directly (vetenquiries@uq.edu.au).

University of Saskatchewan

Applications for admission with advanced standing will only be considered if a vacancy in the Year II class develops. Students applying for advanced standing must meet the normal residency requirements and must be enrolled in a program that has a compatible curriculum. Applicants are required to complete a formal application form and, dependent on their academic record, will be considered for an interview. Part of the interview will be an assessment of their current knowledge. If English is not their first language, applicants will also be required to submit a TOEFL score. Admission is not considered beyond the second year of the program.

APPLICATION AND ENROLLMENT DATA

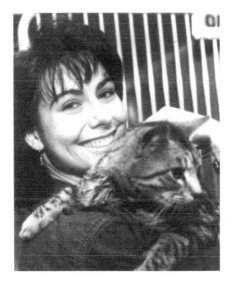

Job satisfaction: giving a little TLC during clinical rounds Photo by Vivian Dixon, courtesy of University of Georgia College of Veterinary Medicine.

Table 1

Applicants to U.S. Colleges of Veterinary Medicine
by Residence, 2004–2013

VMCAS Data Only

Years below represent the year of matriculation

State	2009	2010	2011	2012	2013	AVG
Alabama	105	92	98	98	108	100
Alaska	9	8	9	9	4	8
Alberta	3	0	4	9	9	5
Arizona	85	92	96	88	96	91
Arkansas	35	36	39	42	54	41
Armed Forces (Overseas)	0	0	0	0	2	0
British Columbia	7	5	9	12	14	9
California	655	611	590	657	688	640
Colorado	253	277	251	248	242	254
Connecticut	56	60	56	71	76	64
Delaware	16	10	15	8	11	12
Florida	326	311	322	297	372	326
Foreign	43	43	21	31		35
Georgia	194	189	227	232	259	220
Guam	0	0	0	1	0	0
Hawaii	34	30	25	23	31	29
Idaho	40	23	37	47	43	38
Illinois	249	253	300	241	250	259
Indiana	120	121	137	121	129	126
Iowa	118	139	117	132	120	125
Kansas	130	144	135	101	118	126
Kentucky	91	103	74	94	96	92
Louisiana	148	129	140	156	162	147
Maine	18	31	22	27	22	24
Manitoba	8	4	13	4	1	6
Maryland	130	109	112	141	156	130
Massachusetts	119	106	117	106	120	114
Michigan	241	220	249	212	217	228
Minnesota	182	189	191	169	192	185
Mississippi	70	64	62	78	83	71
Missouri	31	35	40	44	52	40
Washington, DC	6	5	9	7	4	6

Table 1 (continued)

State	2009	2010	2011	2012	2013	AVG
Montana	30	26	26	34	27	29
Nebraska	54	69	59	75	61	64
Nevada	25	24	34	26	35	29
New Brunswick	1	0	0	0	1	0
New Hampshire	21	25	32	28	31	27
New Jersey	115	109	141	160	169	139
New Mexico	36	35	27	36	53	37
New York	263	248	300	313	333	291
Newfoundland & Labrador	0	0	0	0	2	0
North Carolina	225	214	233	216	215	221
North Dakota	23	27	29	23	23	25
Nova Scotia	1	2	3	1	1	2
Ohio	273	304	271	243	274	273
Oklahoma	116	122	109	111	114	114
Ontario	25	20	28	36	26	27
Oregon	99	79	91	103	94	93
Pennsylvania	267	262	250	228	273	256
Prince Edward Island	0	1	1	1	0	1
Province of Quebec	3	3	2	3	6	3
Puerto Rico	29	41	44	39	50	41
Rhode Island	17	18	8	11	12	13
Saskatchewan	4	1	1	1	1	2
South Carolina	85	68	80	70	84	77
South Dakota	18	23	25	26	21	23
Tennessee	169	153	141	132	169	153
Texas	189	213	154	216	256	206
U.S. Territories	0	0	2	0	0	0
Utah	26	31	31	50	55	39
Vermont	11	16	14	16	20	15
Virgin Islands	0	2	2	2	1	1
Virginia	193	176	212	198	196	195
Washington	148	132	141	155	158	147
West Virginia	32	41	32	42	42	38
Wisconsin	175	196	210	187	187	191
Wyoming	13	15	15	17	19	16
Not listed / Not Applicable	0	0	0	0	31	6

Table 2

Applicant Data for Classes 2004–2013

Applications by College

VMCAS Data Only

College Name	2009	2010	2011	2012	2013	AVG
Auburn University	759	667	810	985	1,132	871
Colorado State University	1,877	1,773	1,811	1,576	1,750	1,757
Cornell University	902	868	946	917	1,069	940
Iowa State University	1,043	1,057	1,124	1,182	1,092	1,100
Kansas State University	1,231	1,202	1,342	1,294	1,216	1,257
Louisiana State University	638	667	701	799	699	701
Massey University	152	126	132	105	87	120
Michigan State University	943	902	892	800	894	886
Mississippi State University	760	813	904	899	893	854
Murdoch International	86	85	70	65	58	73
North Carolina State University	553	725	717	662	837	699
Ohio State University	794	792	799	819	1,326	906
Oklahoma State University	452	467	364	655	846	557
Oregon State University	509	455	506	566	854	578
Purdue University	698	674	743	812	767	739
Royal Veterinary College	271	275	125	311	274	251
St. George's University (August Class)	*	*	*	*	534	534
St. George's University (January '14 Class)	*	*	*	*	84	84

Table 2 (continued, college name and years)

College						
University College Dublin	95	170	185	150	155	151
University of California, Davis	1,135	1,057	1,045	1,142	1,136	1,103
University of Edinburgh	195	215	232	257	242	228
University of Florida	871	822	793	748	813	809
University of Georgia	567	551	564	724	843	650
University of Glasgow	224	205	206	194	172	200
University of Guelph-Ontario Veterinary College	85	133	145	136	110	122
University of Illinois	860	781	911	956	989	899
University of Minnesota	1,083	1,025	1,051	949	1,031	1,028
University of Missouri	698	765	913	931	835	828
University of PEI-Atlantic Veterinary College	262	217	223	228	211	228
University of Pennsylvania	1,359	1,209	1,294	1,393	1,533	1,358
University of Tennessee	824	851	730	664	743	762
University of Wisconsin	1,134	1,046	1,196	970	1,219	1,113
Virginia-Maryland Regional College	892	858	967	1,135	1,226	1,016
Washington State University	865	929	1,060	1,061	1,183	1,020
Western University of Health Sciences	754	754	755	769	851	777

* Was not a member of VMCAS in the year indicated.

Table 3

Applicant Data for Classes 2004 - 2013

Age Distribution

VMCAS Data Only

Age	2009	2010	2011	2012	2013	AVG
<20	70	51	46	41	63	54
20	519	486	468	436	463	474
21	1,655	1,729	1,791	1,746	1,903	1765
22	1,116	1,171	1,169	1,131	1,291	1176
23	748	722	780	740	739	746
24	490	524	459	511	500	497
25-30	1,123	1,096	1,045	1,082	1,093	1088
31-35	176	160	198	165	164	173
>30	156	144	124	111	98	127
Other	155	60	185	342	453	239

	2009	2010	2011	2012	2013	
Number of Applicants	6,208	6,032	6,034	5,963	6,769	6,201

Table 4

Applicant Data for Classes 2004 - 2013
Gender Distribution
VMCAS Data Only

	2009 (% of pool)	2010 (% of pool)	2011 (% of pool)	2012 (% of pool)	2013 (% of pool)
Number of Applicants	6,208	6,143	6,265	6,305	6,769
Applicant who identified gender	5,972 (96%)	5,895 (96%)	6,024 (96%)	6,027 (96%)	6,465 (96%)
Total # of Females who identified gender	4,715 (79%)	4,683 (79%)	4,819 (80%)	4,877 (77%)	5,199 (77%)
Total # of Males who identified gender	1,257 (21%)	1,212 (21%)	1,205 (20%)	1,150 (18%)	1,266 (19%)

	2008/2009	2009/2010	2010/2011	2011/2012	2012/2013
Female	.026%	-0.68%	2.90%	1.20%	6.60%
Male	3.88%	-3.58%	-0.58	4.56	10.09

Table 5

Applicant Data for Classes 2009–2013
VMCAS Data Only

	2009	(% response)	2010	(% response)
Number of Applicants	6208		6143	
Number of applicants who responded to at least one race	5778	93.07%	4787	77.93%
Number of applicants who responded to two or more race	3317	53.43%	1356	22.07%
Ethnicity:				
Hispanic - Yes	++	++	374	6.09%
Hispanic - No	++	++	5225	85.06%
Race:				
African-American / Black	135	2.17%	113	1.84%
Spanish / Hispanic / Latino American	335	5.40%	***	***
No Spanish / Hispanic / Latino American	4539	73.12%	***	***
Hispanic American	***	***	***	***
Mexican / Mexican American / Chicano	99	1.59%	***	***
Puerto Rican	72	1.16%	***	***
Cuban	30	0.48%	***	***
Other Spanish / Hispanic / Latino American	122	1.97%	***	***
Other Latino / Spanish American	***	***	***	***
American Indian / Alaskan Native	82	1.32%	115	1.87%
Filipino / Filipino American (Counted as Asian)	31	0.50%	+	+
Chinese / Chinese American (Counted as Asian)	108	1.74%	+	+
Japanese / Japanese American (Counted as Asian)	64	1.03%	+	+
Korean / Korean American (Counted as Asian)	65	1.05%	+	+
Native Hawaiian / Pacific Islander	12	0.19%	25	0.41%
Asian	62	1.00%	315	5.13%
Caucasian / Middle Eastern	4743	76.40%	4319	70.31%
Other	96	1.55%	-	-

Beginning with the VMCAS 2010 cycle, VMCAS has aligned with standard census reporting. As such, there are a number of categories that have been retired (+) and folded into other categories.

   * in 2006 this category choice was moved to the heading of Ethnicity.

   ** was added as a specific ethnicity identifier.

   *** re-categorized under ethnicity.

   ++ Not reported prior to 2010

VMCAS fills between 90% of the seats to Vet Colleges.

VMCAS is seen as representative of the entire pool of applicants.

Table 5 (continued)

Applicant Data for Classes 2009–2013
VMCAS Data Only

	2011	*(% response)*	2012	*(% response)*
Number of Applicants	6265		6305	
Number of applicants who responded to at least one race	4637	74.01%	4908	77.84%
Number of applicants who responded to two or more race	1628	25.99%	187	2.97%
Ethnicity:				
Hispanic - Yes	363	5.79%	409	6.49%
Hispanic - No	5902	94.21%	5296	84.00%
Race:				
African-American / Black	160	2.55%	127	2.01%
Spanish / Hispanic / Latino American	***	***	***	***
No Spanish / Hispanic / Latino American	***	***	***	***
Hispanic American	***	***	***	***
Mexican / Mexican American / Chicano	***	***	***	***
Puerto Rican	***	***	***	***
Cuban	***	***	***	***
Other Spanish / Hispanic / Latino American	***	***	***	***
Other Latino / Spanish American	***	***	***	***
American Indian / Alaskan Native	113	1.80%	69	1.09%
Filipino / Filipino American (Counted as Asian)	+	+	+	+
Chinese / Chinese American (Counted as Asian)	+	+	+	+
Japanese / Japanese American (Counted as Asian)	+	+	+	+
Korean / Korean American (Counted as Asian)	+	+	+	+
Native Hawaiian / Pacific Islander	25	0.40%	18	0.29%
Asian	339	5.41%	263	4.17%
Caucasian / Middle Eastern	4559	72.77%	4431	70.28%
Other	-	-	-	-

Beginning with the VMCAS 2010 cycle, VMCAS has aligned with standard census reporting. As such, there
are a number of categories that have been retired (+) and folded into other categories.

* In 2006 this category choice was moved to the heading of Ethnicity.

** was added as a specific ethnicity identifier.

*** re-categorized under ethnicity.

++ Not reported prior to 2010

VMCAS fills between 90% of the seats to Vet Colleges.

VMCAS is seen as representative of the entire pool of applicants.

Table 5 (continued)
Applicant Data for Classes 2009–2013
VMCAS Data Only

	2013	(% response)
Number of Applicants	6769	
Number of applicants who responded to at least one race	5603	82.77%
Number of applicants who responded to two or more race	262	3.87%

Ethnicity:		
Hispanic - Yes	492	7.27%
Hispanic - No	5631	83.19%

Race:

African-American / Black	177	2.61%
Spanish / Hispanic / Latino American	***	***
No Spanish / Hispanic / Latino American	***	***
Hispanic American	***	***
Mexican / Mexican American / Chicano	***	***
Puerto Rican	***	***
Cuban	***	***
Other Spanish / Hispanic / Latino American	***	***
Other Latino / Spanish American	***	***
American Indian / Alaskan Native	150	2.22%
Filipino / Filipino American (Counted as Asian)	+	+
Chinese / Chinese American (Counted as Asian)	+	+
Japanese / Japanese American (Counted as Asian)	+	+
Korean / Korean American (Counted as Asian)	+	+
Native Hawaiian / Pacific Islander	28	0.41%
Asian	387	5.72%
Caucasian / Middle Eastern	4861	71.81%
Other	-	-

Beginning with the VMCAS 2010 cycle, VMCAS has aligned with standard census reporting. As such, there are a number of categories that have been retired (+) and folded into other categories.

  * in 2006 this category choice was moved to the heading of Ethnicity.

  ** was added as a specific ethnicity identifier.

  *** re-categorized under ethnicity.

  ++ Not reported prior to 2010

VMCAS fills between 90% of the seats to Vet Colleges.

VMCAS is seen as representative of the entire pool of applicants.